# THE
# GASTROPARESIS
# COOKBOOK
# COLLECTION

## ALL THE BEST RECIPES FROM THE GASTROPARESIS COOKBOOK & THE GASTROPARESIS COOKBOOK FOR TWO

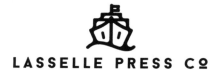

LASSELLE PRESS CO

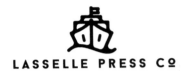

## LASSELLE PRESS C◌

ISBN-13: 978-1911364931
ISBN-10: 1911364936

# CONTENTS

# VEGETARIAN ENTRÉES | 74

# SOUPS & STEWS | 92

## Chapter 9
# SIDES & SNACKS | 114

## Chapter 10
# BROTHS AND CONDIMENTS | 122

## Chapter 11
# SMOOTHIES AND DRINKS | 138

## Chapter 12
# DESSERTS | 150

# CONVERSION CHARTS | 161

# BIBLIOGRAPHY | 162

# INDEX | 163

# INTRODUCTION

Welcome to The Gastroparesis Cookbook Collection.

Here we have combined the best recipes from both The Essential Gastroparesis Cookbook and The Gastroparesis Cookbook For Two. We know that a diagnosis of gastroparesis can be an unpleasant time; it's a chronic condition that can be extremely hard to live with. The good news is that with the right treatments, foods and professional guidance, you can start to feel better again and manage your symptoms effectively.

As well as providing an array of recipes to help control your symptoms, this book is a guide to gastroparesis, including the likely causes, common symptoms and methods of treatment. There are even food lists of ingredients and foods that you can continue to enjoy along with those that you should avoid or cut down. Additionally, the lifestyle hints and tips will hopefully help you feel more confident about getting out and about, and staying healthy and sociable!

Our ultimate aim is to help you enjoy life in the best possible way by eating foods that are right for you, without the constant focus on what you can't eat or do anymore!

We wish you all the best on your journey with gastroparesis.

Happy cooking!

The Lasselle Press Team

# I

# UNDERSTANDING GASTROPARESIS

Whether you have already been diagnosed with gastroparesis, or you've been experiencing uncomfortable symptoms that you think could be gastroparesis, this chapter aims to help by providing information about the condition. Hopefully, it will give you a little more confidence to seek medical advice from your doctor if you haven't already done so. And if you've been diagnosed already, then we hope that this book can provide you with a little more insight and confidence in your decisions about what to eat.

# GASTROPARESIS:

Gastroparesis affects the stomach and the digestive system. When suffering from the condition, your stomach will be less able to digest foods as well as it should do. This can affect your nutrient intake, both due to the problems with the digestion system and because of under-eating/ not being able to consume the same variety of food you may be used to. Unfortunately, gastroparesis usually leads to uncomfortable symptoms in sufferers, especially after eating.

To explain the condition further you will need to know a little more about the stomach: the stomach muscles usually work to contract and digest food before passing this digested food through to the intestines, and ultimately out of the body. Both solids and liquids are processed in this way and are broken down into tiny particles. Thus, liquids and soft foods are always easier to digest than solids as they start as smaller particles to begin with.

For those suffering with gastroparesis, the stomach muscles do not work in the way that they should do, which is usually caused by damage to the vagus nerve. This nerve is responsible for controlling the stomach muscles' movements and contractions. As a result of poor muscle movement and slow digestion, the food is not broken down as it should be. This delays the stomach from emptying and so food can remain there for long periods of time, and in some cases, stay there. This can lead to further problems such as bacteria growth in the stomach and bezoars.

# CAUSES OF GASTROPARESIS:

There are a variety of potential causes of gastroparesis. In certain individuals, the cause is unknown (idiopathic) and cannot be pinned down to any one factor. However, other possible causes are outlined below:

DIABETES TYPE 1 AND TYPE 2: If uncontrolled and sugar levels are not regulated, this can lead to gastroparesis.

ABDOMINAL SURGERY THAT INJURES THE VAGUS NERVE: Often a complication of gastric bypass surgery.

CERTAIN MEDICATIONS: Including certain tricyclic antidepressants, calcium channel blockers and narcotics, nicotine, progesterone, lithium and clonidine (always speak to your doctor if unsure).

HORMONAL DISORDERS (ENDOCRINE): Addison's disease, hyperparathyroidism, hypothyroidism, or hormone imbalance. Consult your doctor if you have any of these and notice the symptoms outlined in the next chapter.

AUTOIMMUNE DISEASES: Parkinson's, multiple sclerosis and others (controlling inflammation is really important here). Consult your doctor if you have any of these and notice the symptoms outlined in the next chapter.

EATING DISORDERS: Anorexia and Bulimia. It is important to consider that you may suffer from gastroparesis if you are suffering, or have suffered, one of these disorders. Again, consult your doctor if you experience any unusual symptoms.

# SYMPTOMS:

The following symptoms may be an indicator of gastroparesis. Please consult your doctor to discuss these symptoms:

- Heartburn,
- Nausea,
- Stomach pain,
- Vomiting undigested food,
- Feeling full very quickly after eating,
- Bloating of the abdominal cavity,
- Weight loss and a loss of appetite,
- Fluctuating blood sugar levels - particularly problematic for those with diabetes,
- Bacteria growth on the stomach lining, leading to bacterial infections in the body (this would need to be diagnosed by a professional).

These symptoms may not necessarily indicate gastroparesis and may be symptoms of other illnesses or diseases, so you should always consult a professional for a diagnosis. Likewise, it could be that these symptoms are a result of gastroparesis as well as another disease or illness. If you're suffering from a known disease but notice these symptoms, or anything out of the ordinary, you must see your doctor.

# TREATING GASTROPARESIS:

Eating a healthy and controlled diet can help control the symptoms of gastroparesis but cannot cure or treat it alone. It is crucial that a healthcare professional diagnose this condition and offer support and medication as well as dietary and lifestyle advice; there are also procedures that can help with emptying the stomach. This book should be used as a guide alongside this information and aims to provide you with recommended dietary choices as well as recipes to try out in the kitchen. It is also important to take into consideration, any other dietary restrictions you may have as a result of other conditions including diabetes, celiac disease, or lactose intolerance.

Alongside your diet, you may find that changes to your lifestyle will have a positive impact on your symptoms. Consider the following:

1. Exercise: it is recommended that you exercise for at least 20-30 minutes per day. This can be either a walk, jog, yoga, or even something a little more strenuous.
2. Drink plenty of water: this will not only keep you hydrated but will aid the digestive system.
3. Sleep: try and get 8 hours sleep per night.
4. Posture: sit upright as much as you can, in particular when relaxing. It is important to find a chair that will help with this posture in order to help the digestive system. After meals, stay sitting upright or try to go for a light walk.

# II

# DIET AND NUTRITION TIPS FOR GASTROPARESIS

This chapter will outline different dietary and lifestyle changes you can consider making to help you control your gastroparesis and the symptoms that come with it. Different types of 'diet' that you may consider are also outlined lists of foods that you can continue to enjoy as well as those that you should avoid or cut down on are given.

# RECOMMENDATIONS FOR THE GASTROPARESIS DIET:

- Liquids are easier to digest than solids so make the most of wholesome broths and soups as well as shakes, particularly when your symptoms flare up.
- Eating little and often is far better than eating big portions. Aim for 5-6 small meals a day rather than 3 big ones.
- Aim to consume less than 40g fat per day. If you're eating 6 meals per day then your fat intake should be 6-7g per meal.
- Thoroughly chew each mouthful to give your stomach a hand! Soft, ground, strained or puréed foods are easier to digest than solids.
- FODMAPS - consider restricting FODMAPS (more information in the next section).
- Avoid red meat.
- Eat and drink separately.
- Lower your fiber intake - especially whole grains, raw fruit and vegetables with skins, and wheat.
- Avoid foods high in fructose and polyols (artificial sweeteners like sorbitol).
- Take a walk or ensure you sit upright after eating (for at least one hour) in order to aid the digestion process.
- Peel fruit and vegetables before blending, cooking or straining.
- Low fat dairy options are advised - some milk products may flare up symptoms, so it is important that you monitor your reactions to these and choose dairy-free alternatives if lactose intolerant.
- Given that you are going to need to lower your fat, fiber and sugar intake, it can sometimes be difficult to meet your daily nutritional needs. Speak to your doctor or dietitian about supplementing your diet with multivitamins such as B6, B12, fish oils etc. This will depend on the vitamins you are lacking from the foods you are reducing or avoiding. Other than multivitamins, shakes and smoothies are a great way of consuming vitamins.

# OTHER DIETARY CONSIDERATIONS

FODMAPS (Fermentable Oligosaccharides, Disaccharides, Monosaccharides and Polyols)

These are simple and complex sugars that are poorly absorbed after food has been digested. They are found in a variety of fruits, vegetables, milk, and wheat. They pass through the stomach and the small intestine without changing state and are then fermented by colonic bacteria, resulting in a release of gas; or they are expelled from the body with fluids. The retention of these sugars often leads to bloating, abdominal pain and diarrhoea, particularly for those with sensitive stomachs and IBS. For some with gastroparesis, FODMAPS can make digestion even harder. Please note that your reaction to these types of foods vary between patients, and these are suggestions to the types of foods you could consider monitoring.

FODMAP foods to avoid include:
* Onion, garlic, pulses, brassicas (cauliflower, broccoli, cabbage etc.),
* Wheat,
* Fruit e.g. plums, peaches, nectarines, apples and other stoned fruits,
* Lactose (for those who are lactose intolerant).


Diabetes

If you have diabetes and gastroparesis, this can be extremely confusing and difficult to manage. The major consideration here is controlling your blood sugar levels. This can be done through insulin as well as your diet. Meals should be kept small and eaten at regular times. You should continue to eat carbohydrates in equal proportions for each meal to help regulate your blood sugar levels. It is recommended that you consume between 30-40g carbohydrates per meal and eat 6 meals per day. You should be consuming between 210-240g carbohydrates per day depending on your gender and size and what your doctor has recommended. Speak to a professional if unsure.

## Gluten-Free

For some, going gluten-free can help control symptoms of gastroparesis. For those suffering from celiac disease or gluten allergies this is essential.

## Dairy-Free

Lactose in dairy products can flare up symptoms for some, and if you're lactose intolerant, need avoiding. In this case, just substitute any dairy items in the recipes with dairy free. We've included a great almond milk and rice milk recipe to use too!

## GERD friendly

Gastroesophageal reflux disease can cause uncomfortable symptoms such as heartburn and is caused by different foods which range from one person to another. Common foods that flare symptoms are tomatoes, citrus, spices and chocolate.

# FOODS TO ADD TO YOUR SHOPPING LIST:

Ginger ale
Fat-free soups
Bouillon soups
Saltine crackers
Skim milk
Skim milk products
Low-fat Greek yogurt
Low-fat cheese
Fat free soups
Fat-free broths
Vegetable soups
White bread, rice or pasta
Eggs (limit egg yolks)
Peanut butter (up to 2 tbsp per day)
Vegetable juices
Beets
Carrots
Mushrooms
Spinach
Summer squash
Acorn squash
Strained tomato sauce
Yams
Apple juice
Grape juice
Pineapple juice
Cranberry juice
Coconut oil
Frozen yogurt
Gelatin
Jelly
Skinless chicken and turkey breasts
Ground lean chicken and turkey
Soft fish e.g. sea bass, cod, haddock
Apple sauce
Skinless peaches and pears

Sparkling water
Margarines and butters (in small amounts)
Low-fat mayonnaise
Gluten free foods
Gluten free pasta and bread
White bread
Canned fruits (skinless)
Extra virgin olive oil
Egg noodles
Rice cakes
Honey
Maple syrup
Green tea
Tea
Gatorade

Stock your pantry with:
Dried herbs: thyme, basil, sage, tarragon, parsley etc.
Dried spices: cinnamon, ground nutmeg, ground ginger, cloves

# FOODS TO AVOID:

Whole milk products
Creams
Soups that are made with cream or whole milk
Fatty broths
Fruits with skin on and dried fruits
Steak and red meat
Peas
Dried beans
Lentils
Oatmeal
Cereal
Whole grain rice
Whole grain bread
Raw vegetables
Green beans, wax, and Lima beans with skins
Brussels spouts
Cauliflower
Corn
Cabbage
Celery

Onion
Peppers
Eggplant
Turnips
Sauerkraut
Water chestnuts
Desserts high in fat, such as cakes, cookies, ice cream, pies, or pastries
Fruit preservatives
Packaged and processed foods
Cayenne pepper

# III
# EATING OUT AND SHOPPING GUIDE

You'll still want to eat out even when you have to be careful with your food. This chapter aims to provide you with some hints and tips to make this easier.

# TIPS FOR EATING OUT:

After receiving a diagnosis of gastroparesis, or even before, you may have found the idea or experience of eating out quite intimidating. Just one look at the menu and all those rich, fatty food options probably send your mind straight to the thought of pain and flare ups. It can be an uncomfortable, if not distressing time, but having gastroparesis needn't mean you can't enjoy eating out with friends and family.

- Suggest a restaurant to friends and family once you've browsed their menu and made sure that there is at least one dish on there that would be suitable for you to order.
- Consider calling the restaurant beforehand to explain the types of foods you can and can't have. Those working in this industry will usually be more than happy to cater for specific dietary needs and if they're not, they're not worth your custom!
- Ask for dishes to be cooked in olive oil rather than butter or vegetable oils.
- Opt for seafood or poultry options and ask how they're cooked.
- Drink before or after your meal and not during.
- Ask about small or half portions and order these.
- Don't let yourself go hungry before you go out; work out if this is going to be the last meal of the day and if so have your other meals beforehand. If it's lunchtime, ensure you have eaten enough meals beforehand and that you will be able to eat the rest of your meals afterwards.

# TRAVELING:

It may be difficult to go out for the whole day, let alone the weekend, week, or even longer! The thought of not having foods available to you can be daunting; you really wouldn't want to find yourself in the position of grabbing something from the shop or café, just because you're hungry and in a rush.

Prep your meals for the day and store them in containers. If you're not going to be somewhere with a microwave, ensure these can be eaten cold and straight from the container. If you're staying away, you could always take extra portions for the next day and ask the hotel to store them for you and even heat them up.

It's also worth researching the restaurants and cafés where you are visiting and following the advice given for eating out. Creating a meal plan for the duration of your stay is a good idea, so that you are not left in a tricky situation. Finally, taking pre-made shakes and smoothies is a great way to consume your calories whilst on the move.

# GROCERY SHOPPING:

1. Always write a list and check it against the recommended foods as well as those that are not allowed.
2. Plan out your meals so that you know exactly how much of each item you need.
3. Check out the reduced items section to see what bargains you can get your hands on!
4. Ask your family to support you and try similar foods to you, so that you don't have temptations lying around the kitchen. Obviously they will need to eat a different diet to you and bigger portions, but they could try and stick to foods such as poultry and seafood instead of red meats and fatty foods.
5. Don't grocery shop on an empty stomach - you'll only find yourself tempted by snacks and convenient foods.

# IV

# GETTING STARTED

In order to help you get started on this diet, there are a few things that you will need to be able to prepare the foods and meals in this cookbook.

# KITCHEN EQUIPMENT

- Blender/ food processor
- Crock pot, pots, skillet
- Steam basket/steamer/colander
- Oven dish, tray
- Potato masher
- Large mixing bowls
- Foil/plastic wrap
- Tupperware boxes
- Stocking your cupboard:
- Ensure you purchase a variety of dry ingredients that can be used to add flavor to your foods (see foods to enjoy list).

# KEEPING A FOOD JOURNAL

It is always a good idea to keep a record of the foods and drinks you consume as well as your symptoms. This way you can track when your symptoms flare up and what may have caused them to do so. In the same way, if you're working to cut out a certain food group at a time, this is a great method for seeing if it makes a difference, as well as if there are certain foods that you know you should avoid. Like any condition, each person experiences gastroparesis differently, and while some foods will be okay for one person, they may be intolerable for others. Keep a journal and use this alongside your doctor's recommendations and these recipes, to work out what's best for you.

Now that you have all you need to know to get your kitchen stocked with the right foods and equipment; you've planned out how many meals you need a day; and you know what you can eat - you're ready to go! The gastroparesis road can be long and taxing but hopefully with the following recipes and a lot of self-love and encouragement, you will be able to control your symptoms as best as possible, continue to enjoy meal times, and feel happier and healthier again.

# BREAKFAST

# ACORN SQUASH PANCAKES

**SERVES 2 / PREP TIME: 3 MINUTES / COOK TIME: 40 MINUTES**

These pancakes will keep you going until your next meal and taste delicious.

---

**1/4 CUP ACORN SQUASH, PEELED AND CHOPPED**

**2 EGG WHITES**

**1 TSP OREGANO**

**A PINCH OF SEA SALT**

**1 TSP OLIVE OIL**

---

1. Bring a pot of water to boil over a high heat.
2. Add the chopped acorn squash, reduce the heat and simmer for 30-40 minutes or until very soft.
3. Drain.
4. Allow squash to cool slightly and blend in a food processor until puréed.
5. Whisk together the egg whites, oregano, puréed squash and sea salt in a mixing bowl.
6. Heat the olive oil in a pan over a medium heat.
7. Pour 1/2 the batter into the pan and cook for 4-5 minutes.
8. Flip over and allow to cook on the other side for 1-2 minutes.
9. Repeat for the second pancake.
10. Serve with your choice of sweet accompaniment (honey or maple syrup) or alone for a savory breakfast.

Per serving: Calories: 54; Fat: 3g (Saturated Fat: 1g); Carbohydrates: 3g; Fiber: 0.5g; Sugar: 0g; Sodium: 385mg; Protein: 6g

# BANANA PANCAKES

**SERVES 2 / PREP TIME: 5 MINUTES / COOK TIME: 5 MINUTES**

Pancakes work wonders for one of your small meals a day.

---

**1 VERY RIPE SMALL BANANA**

**2 LARGE EGG WHITES**

**1/2 CUP NON-FAT GREEK YOGURT**

---

1. Blend all the ingredients in a food processor until smooth.
2. Heat a non-stick skillet over a medium heat.
3. Pour batter into pancake shapes and cook for 1-2 minutes on each side.
4. Enjoy!

Per serving: Calories: 133; Fat:0g (Saturated Fat: 0g); Carbohydrates: 17g; Fiber: 1g; Sugar: 11g; Sodium: 164mg; Protein: 17g

# MATCHA CHICKEN BROTH

**SERVES 4 / PREP TIME: 5 MINUTES / COOK TIME: 40 MINUTES**

This unusual blend of flavors really hits the spot.

---

**2 CUPS LOW SODIUM CHICKEN STOCK**

**2 CUPS WATER**

**1 CUP POTATOES, PEELED AND CHOPPED**

**1 CUP SPINACH**

**1 TSP MATCHA GREEN TEA POWDER**

---

1. Add the chicken stock and water to a pan over a medium-high heat.
2. Once bubbling (but not boiling), lower the heat slightly and add the potatoes, spinach and matcha powder.
3. Leave to simmer for 30-35 minutes or until potatoes are very soft.
4. Allow to cool slightly before blending in a food processor.
5. Stir and serve immediately.

Per serving: Calories: 101; Fat: 2.5g (Saturated Fat: 0g); Carbohydrates: 6.5g; Fiber: 1.5g; Sugar: 0.3g; Sodium: 207mg; Protein: 3.3g

# APPLE CREAM OF WHEAT BREAKFAST

**SERVES 2 / PREP TIME: 5 MINUTES / COOK TIME: 5 MINUTES**

A scrumptious warm porridge.

---

**1 CUP SKIM MILK**

**1/2 CUP WATER**

**1/2 CUP CREAM OF WHEAT**

**1/4 CUP APPLE SAUCE**

**1 TSP CINNAMON**

---

1. Bring the milk and water to the boil in a pot and reduce to a simmer.
2. Stir in the cream of wheat until the sauce starts to thicken (over a low heat).
3. Leave to simmer for 2-3 minutes, then stir in the apple sauce and cinnamon.
4. Serve hot!

Per serving: Calories: 88; Fat: 0g (Saturated Fat: 0g); Carbohydrates: 16g; Fiber: 1.5g; Sugar: 8g; Sodium: 150mg; Protein: 5g

# TURKEY BROTH

**SERVES 2 / PREP TIME: 5 MINUTES / COOK TIME: 35 MINUTES**

Can be enjoyed for a warming breakfast or throughout the day.

---

| | |
|---|---|
| **4OZ SKINLESS, BONELESS TURKEY BREAST** | **1/4 CUP ACORN SQUASH, PEELED AND CHOPPED** |
| **1/2 CUP CHICKEN STOCK** | **1 TSP DRIED THYME** |
| **1 CUP WATER** | **1 TSP DRIED SAGE** |

---

1. Bring a large pot of water to the boil over a high heat.
2. Add the turkey breast meat and poach in the water over a medium heat for 10-15 minutes or until cooked throughout and not pink.
3. Meanwhile, cook your squash by steaming over the pot for the same amount of time as the turkey (make sure these are extremely soft).
4. Remove the turkey and squash once cooked.
5. Slice the turkey breast.
6. Into a new pan add all of the ingredients and bring to the boil over a high heat.
7. Lower the heat and allow to simmer for 10-15 minutes.
8. Serve right away!

Tip: If you need to Purée your vegetables, simply blend the whole broth in a food processor until completely smooth.

Per serving: Calories: 79; Fat: 2g (Saturated Fat: 0g); Carbohydrates: 3g; Fiber: 1g; Sugar: 0; Sodium: 43mg; Protein: 14g; Potassium: 262mg

# WAFFLES WITH PURÉED PEACHES

**SERVES 4 / PREP TIME: 10 MINUTES / COOK TIME: 15 MINUTES**

A sweet-tooth's favorite!

---

1 CUP GLUTEN-FREE FLOUR

2 TSP BAKING POWDER

1 TSP CINNAMON

A PINCH OF SEA SALT

1 CUP SKIM MILK

2 TBSP LEMON JUICE

1 LARGE BANANA, CRUSHED WITH A FORK

2 TSP VANILLA EXTRACT

1 CUP CANNED PEACHES (SKINLESS)

---

1. Preheat oven to 275°F/140 °C/Gas Mark 1.
2. Whisk the flour, baking powder, cinnamon and salt together.
3. In a separate bowl, whisk the milk, lemon juice, banana and the vanilla together.
4. Mix the dry ingredients into the wet.
5. Heat up a waffle maker and pour the waffle batter to make 4 waffles for 10-15 minutes each or until cooked through.
6. Meanwhile, heat a pan over a low heat and add the peaches for 5-10 minutes or until warmed through. Whiz in a food processor if peaches are still too chunky.
7. Serve the waffles with the peach sauce and enjoy.

Per serving: Calories: 130; Fat: 1g (Saturated Fat: 0g); Carbohydrates: 30g; Fiber: 0g; Sugar: 13g; Sodium: 98mg; Protein: 3g

# CHIVE & SPINACH FRITTATA

**SERVES 4  /  PREP TIME: 5 MINUTES  /  COOK TIME: 8 MINUTES**

An easy to prepare, delicious breakfast.

---

6 EGG WHITES

1 TBSP CHOPPED CHIVES

1 TSP DRIED THYME

1 CUP FROZEN SPINACH, THAWED

1 TBSP GREEK YOGURT (FAT FREE)

1 TSP OLIVE OIL

---

1. Preheat the broiler on a low heat.
2. Whisk the eggs, chives, thyme, spinach and Greek yogurt together.
3. Pour the mixture into a lightly oiled shallow baking dish/oven-proof skillet.
4. Place under the broiler for 6-8 minutes or until cooked through.
5. Slice and enjoy.

Per serving: Calories: 40; Fat: 1g (Saturated Fat: 0g); Carbohydrates: 3g; Fiber: 2g; Sugar: 1g; Sodium: 184mg; Protein: 7g

# SMASHED SPINACH AND SCRAMBLED EGGS

**SERVES 4 / PREP TIME: 2 MINUTES / COOK TIME: 8 MINUTES**

A simple yet special breakfast.

---

1 TSP UNSALTED BUTTER/OLIVE OIL

4 EGG WHITES

1 TBSP SKIM MILK OR EQUIVALENT

1/4 CUP CANNED SPINACH

4 SLICES GLUTEN-FREE BREAD

1 TSP PARSLEY, CHOPPED

---

1. Heat a skillet over medium heat and add the butter/oil.
2. Whisk the eggs with the milk and add to the skillet.
3. Lower the heat slightly and continue to whisk for 4-5 minutes for soft eggs. Continue to stir for a couple more minutes if you like them more firm.
4. Add the spinach for 1-2 minutes over a low heat and allow to wilt.
5. Meanwhile add the bread to the toaster.
6. Once the toast is golden, top with the scrambled eggs.
7. Sprinkle with parsley and a squeeze of lemon juice if desired.
8. Enjoy!

Per serving: Calories: 102; Fat: 3g (Saturated Fat: 1g); Carbohydrates: 14g; Fiber: 2g; Sugar: 2g; Sodium: 232mg; Protein: 7g

# RASPBERRY PANCAKES

**SERVES 6 / PREP TIME: 5 MINUTES / COOK TIME: 5 MINUTES**

The raspberries turn these pancakes a lovely deep purple and taste amazing!

| | |
|---|---|
| 1 TSP UNSALTED BUTTER/OLIVE OIL | 1 CUP WHITE FLOUR (GF IF NEEDED) |
| 1 CUP CANNED RASPBERRIES, SKINLESS | 1 TSP BAKING POWDER |
| 3 TBSP HONEY | 2 EGGS |
| 1 CUP GREEK YOGURT (FAT-FREE) | |

1. Add all the wet ingredients (except eggs) to a bowl and whisk.
2. Add the dry ingredients to a separate bowl and mix.
3. Pour the wet ingredients into the dry and whisk until combined.
4. Beat the eggs.
5. Fold the eggs into the batter.
6. Heat a skillet over a medium heat and then add 1/6 of the mixture to form a pancake.
7. Cook for 2 minutes each side or until cooked through and golden.
8. Repeat with the mixture (keep an oven on a low heat to make sure the cooked pancakes stay warm whilst you're doing the rest).
9. Serve with a little extra Greek yogurt.

Per serving: Calories: 173; Fat: 2g (Saturated Fat: 1g); Carbohydrates: 30g; Fiber: 2g; Sugar: 12g; Sodium: 164mg; Protein: 9g

# BEET OMELET

**SERVES 2  /  PREP TIME: 5 MINUTES  /  COOK TIME: 10 MINUTES**

This is a fast and fresh breakfast that can be cooked up in advance.

---

**3 EGG WHITES**

**2 TBSP CHOPPED CHIVES**

**1 TSP DRIED BASIL**

**1 TBSP FAT FREE GREEK YOGURT**

**1 TSP OLIVE OIL**

**1/4 CUP CANNED BEETS, SLICED**

---

1. Preheat the broiler/grill on a low heat.
2. Whisk the eggs, chives, basil and Greek yogurt together.
3. Pour the mixture into a lightly oiled shallow baking dish/oven-proof skillet.
4. Layer the top of the frittata with the sliced beets.
5. Cook for 5-6 minutes or until cooked through.
6. Gently lift the edges with a spatula and flip over. Cook for a further 2 minutes and serve.

Per serving: Calories: 57; Fat: 2g (Saturated Fat: 0g); Carbohydrates: 3g; Fiber: 1g; Sugar: 2g; Sodium: 204mg; Protein: 7g

# CHERRY CREAM OF RICE CEREAL

**SERVES 4 / PREP TIME: 5 MINUTES   COOK TIME: 10 MINUTES**

Warm and wholesome!

---

1 CUP UNCOOKED WHITE RICE

2 CUPS PINEAPPLE JUICE

2 CUPS WATER

1/2 CUP SKIM MILK

2 TBSP PURE HONEY

1 TSP VANILLA EXTRACT

1 TSP NUTMEG

1 CUP CANNED CHERRIES (PITTED & SKINLESS)

---

1. Blend the rice in a food processor or grinder until it is a fine powder.
2. Add the juice, water, milk, honey, nutmeg and vanilla extract to a pan over a high heat until it reaches a boil.
3. Gradually add the rice to the pan whilst stirring.
4. Turn down the heat and cover.
5. Allow to simmer for 5 minutes.
6. Add the canned cherries for an additional 3 minutes or until hot through.
7. Stir before serving.

Per serving: Calories: 197; Fat: 0g (Saturated Fat: 0g); Carbohydrates: 47g; Fiber: 1g; Sugar: 30g; Sodium: 18mg; Protein: 3g

# GASTROPARESIS BREAKFAST SMOOTHIE

**SERVES 2 / PREP TIME: 5 MINUTES / COOK TIME: NA**

Tropical flavours!

---

**1/2 CUP GREEK YOGURT (FAT-FREE)**

**1/2 PEELED BANANA, FRESH OR FROZEN**

**1/4 CUP CANNED PEACHES, SKINLESS**

**1/2 TSP NUTMEG**

---

1. Blend all ingredients in a smoothie maker until there are no lumps left.
2. Serve over crushed ice!
3. Sprinkle over a little extra nutmeg over the top if desired.

Hint: If you need to, strain the smoothie through a muslin cloth or sieve to get rid of any little bits that may be left from the fruit.

Per serving: Calories: 243; Fat: 1g (Saturated Fat: 1g); Carbohydrates: 34g; Fiber: 2g; Sugar: 26g; Sodium: 119mg; Protein: 27g

# RICE PUFF BIRCHER

SERVES 2  /  PREP TIME: 5 MINUTES / COOK TIME: 30 MINUTES

Delicious smooth and crispy contrast!

---

1/2 CUP CANNED PEARS, SKINLESS &
UNSWEETENED

1 TSP NUTMEG

1 TSP CINNAMON

1 TSP STEVIA

1 CUP WATER

1 CUP NON-FAT GREEK YOGURT

1/2 CUP RICE PUFF CEREAL (RICE
KRISPIES TM)

---

1. Add the pears, nutmeg, cinnamon, stevia and water to a pan over a high heat and bring to almost boiling point.
2. Reduce the heat, cover and simmer for 20-30 minutes or until reduced.
3. Remove from the pan and allow to cool.
4. Stir the rice puff cereal into the yogurt and then stir in the pear compote.
5. Cover and refrigerate overnight for a delicious bircher-style breakfast in the morning!

Hint: Alternatively serve the compote warm for a contrast in temperatures!

Per serving: Calories: 124; Fat: 1g (Saturated Fat: 0g); Carbohydrates: 18g; Fiber: 2g; Sugar: 10g; Sodium: 93mg; Protein: 14g

# CHIVE & POTATO CAKES

**SERVES 4 / PREP TIME: 15 MINUTES / COOK TIME: 20 MINUTES**

Sublime!

---

**2 PEELED AND DICED WHITE POTATOES**

**2 TBSP CUP CHIVES**

**A PINCH OF SALT**

**2 TBSP NON-FAT FAT GREEK YOGURT**

**2 TSP UNSALTED BUTTER/OLIVE OIL**

---

1. Bring a full pot of water to the boil over a high heat.
2. Add potatoes, lower heat slightly and allow to simmer for 10-15 minutes until soft.
3. Drain and remove from the pan.
4. Use a potato masher to mash potatoes in a mixing bowl and add chives, salt and yogurt before mixing well.
5. Use your hands to shape the potato mixture into two patties.
6. Now melt the unsalted butter/oil in a skillet over a medium heat.
7. Add each hash brown to the skillet and brown each side for 3-4 minutes.

Per serving: Calories: 36; Fat: 2g (Saturated Fat: 1.5g); Carbohydrates: 3.5g; Fiber: 0.5g; Sugar: 0.5g; Sodium: 5mg; Protein: 1.5g

# GREEK YOGURT & HOMEMADE FRUIT COMPOTE

**SERVES 4 / PREP TIME: 5 MINUTES / COOK TIME: 30 MINUTES**

Pre-prepare the compote and store in a sealed container before simply adding to Greek yogurt!

---

1 CUP CANNED PEARS (SKINLESS)

1 TSP GROUND NUTMEG

1 TSP CINNAMON

1 TSP STEVIA POWDER

1 CUP WATER

1 CUP GREEK YOGURT (FAT-FREE)

---

1. Add the drained fruit, spices and water to a pan over a high heat and bring to almost boiling point.
2. Reduce the heat, cover and simmer for 20-30 minutes or until reduced and lovely and thick.
3. Can be served warm over the Greek yogurt or cool.

Per serving: Calories: 78; Fat: 0g (Saturated Fat: 0g); Carbohydrates: 14g; Fiber: 2g; Sugar: 11g; Sodium: 31mg; Protein: 7g

# CHICKEN PATTIES

**SERVES 4 / PREP TIME: 5 MINUTES / COOK TIME: 12 MINUTES**

A meaty breakfast - great for the weekends!

---

**8OZ GROUND CHICKEN BREAST**

**1/2 MEDIUM CARROT, PEELED AND GRATED**

**1 TSP DRIED TARRAGON**

**1 TBSP WATER**

**1 TBSP OLIVE OIL**

---

1. Mix all the ingredients in a large bowl (save the oil for cooking).
2. Using wet hands, create 4 patties from the chicken mixture.
3. Heat the oil in a skillet over a medium heat.
4. Cook the patties for 5-6 minutes on each side or until thoroughly cooked through.
5. Serve!

Per serving: Calories: 58; Fat: 4g (Saturated Fat: 1g); Carbohydrates: 1g; Fiber: 0g; Sugar: 0g; Sodium: 77mg; Protein: 4g

# MUSHROOM CRACKERS

**SERVES 4 / PREP TIME: 5 MINUTES / COOK TIME: 10 MINUTES**

Add a bit of variety to the boring dry crackers you may be used to.

---

**1 TSP OLIVE OIL**

**1 CUP MUSHROOMS**

**1 TSP DRIED THYME**

**1 TSP DRIED BASIL**

**4 PLAIN SALTINE CRACKERS**

---

1. Heat the oil in a skillet over a medium heat and add the mushrooms and herbs.
2. Sauté for 10 minutes until thoroughly cooked.
3. Serve the mushrooms on each cracker.
4. Enjoy.

Per serving: Calories: 18; Fat: 0g (Saturated Fat: 0g); Carbohydrates: 3g; Fiber: 0g; Sugar: 0g; Sodium: 30mg; Protein: 1g

# PEACH CRÊPES

**SERVES 2 / PREP TIME: 5 MINUTES / COOK TIME: 15 MINUTES**

Sweet and scrumptious!

---

1 TBSP HONEY

1/4 CUP NON-FAT GREEK YOGURT

1 EGG YOLK

1/3 CUP WHITE FLOUR (GLUTEN-FREE IF NEEDED)

1/2 TSP BAKING POWDER

1 EGG WHITE

1 TSP UNSALTED BUTTER

1/4 CUP CANNED PEACHES, SKINLESS

---

1. Heat the peaches in a skillet over a medium heat for 4-5 minutes to warm through.
2. Blend in a food processor to purée and place to one side.
3. Whisk the honey, Greek yogurt and egg yolk in a bowl.
4. Add the dry ingredients to a separate bowl and mix.
5. Gradually add the wet ingredients into the dry, whilst whisking until combined.
6. Now beat the egg white into soft peaks.
7. Fold the egg white into the batter.
8. Heat a skillet over a medium heat and melt the butter.
9. Pour 1/2 of the mixture in the skillet to form a pancake.
10. Cook for 2 minutes on each side or until cooked through and golden.
11. Repeat with the rest of the mixture.
12. Serve each crêpe with the puréed peach and a little sugar if desired.

Per serving: Calories: 226; Fat: 5g (Saturated Fat: 2g); Carbohydrates: 28g; Fiber: 1g; Sugar: 8g; Sodium: 267mg; Protein: 18g; Potassium: 278mg

# CHEESE & PINEAPPLE BRUNCH

**SERVES 2 / PREP TIME: 5 MINUTES / COOK TIME: 10 MINUTES**

A fruity-cheesy accompaniment to your usual crackers!

---

**1/4 CUP CANNED PINEAPPLE (UN-SWEETENED), DICED**

**1/2 CUP LOW FAT COTTAGE CHEESE**

**2 SALTINE CRACKERS**

---

1. Sauté the pineapple in a skillet over a medium heat for 10 minutes.
2. Remove and allow to cool completely.
3. Mix together with the cottage cheese.
4. Serve with the crackers on the side for a healthy and filling brunch or snack.

Per serving: Calories: 71; Fat: 2g (Saturated Fat: 1g); Carbohydrates: 7g; Fiber: 0g; Sugar: 4g; Sodium: 215mg; Protein: 7g

# CRANBERRY RICE PUDDING

**SERVES 2 / PREP TIME: 5 MINUTES   COOK TIME: 10 MINUTES**

So creamy and sweet!

---

1/2 CUP UNCOOKED WHITE RICE

1/4 CUP APPLE JUICE

1/2 CUP WATER

1/4 CUP RICE MILK

1 TBSP PURE HONEY

1 TSP GROUND NUTMEG

1 TSP VANILLA EXTRACT

1/2 CUP CANNED CRANBERRIES, SKIN-LESS (OR ALTERNATIVE CANNED FRUIT OF CHOICE)

---

1.  Blend the rice in a food processor or grinder until powdered.
2.  Add the juice, water, rice milk, honey, nutmeg and vanilla extract to a pan over a high heat and bring to the boil.
3.  Gradually add the rice powder to the pan whilst stirring.
4.  Turn down the heat and cover to simmer for 5 minutes.
5.  Add the canned cranberries for 3 minutes or until hot through.
6.  Stir before serving.

Per serving: Calories: 173; Fat: 1g (Saturated Fat: 0g); Carbohydrates: 40g; Fiber: 1g; Sugar: 27g; Sodium: 32mg; Protein: 1g; Potassium: 82mg

# BREAKFAST BANANA MUFFINS

**SERVES 2 / PREP TIME: 10 MINUTES / COOK TIME: 18 MINUTES**

Delightful muffins to start your day!

---

2 TBSP NON-FAT SOUR CREAM

1/2 TSP VANILLA EXTRACT

1/2 TBSP CANOLA OIL

1 LARGE EGG WHITE

1/2 CUP WHITE FLOUR (GLUTEN-FREE IF NEEDED)

1/2 TSP BAKING POWDER

1 SMALL RIPE BANANA, PEELED AND SLICED

---

1. Preheat oven to 400°F/200 °C/Gas Mark 6.
2. Line a muffin tray with 4 muffin cases or lightly oil.
3. In a small bowl combine sour cream, vanilla extract, oil and egg white.
4. In a larger bowl, mix the dry ingredients together.
5. Now stir the wet ingredients into the dry ingredients.
6. Mix in the sliced banana.
7. Divide the batter into 4 muffin cases and then bake in the oven for 15-18 minutes or until cooked through.
8. Enjoy alone!

Hint: These muffins are great to pop in a lunch box for a breakfast on the go!

Per serving: Calories: 182; Fat:1g (Saturated Fat: 0g); Carbohydrates: 38g; Fiber: 2g; Sugar: 7g; Sodium: 198mg; Protein: 6g; Potassium: 263mg

# SEAFOOD & POULTRY

# CHICKEN, CARROT & ZUCCHINI NOODLES

**SERVES 4 / PREP TIME: 5 MINUTES / COOK TIME: 20 MINUTES**

A simple yet scrumptious entrée.

---

**1/2 CUP CARROTS, PEELED, GRATED & STEAMED**

**1/2 CUP ZUCCHINI, PEELED, GRATED & STEAMED**

**1 TBSP COCONUT OIL**

**8OZ CHICKEN BREASTS, SKINLESS AND GROUND**

**1 CUP EGG NOODLES, COOKED**

**1 TSP ALLSPICE**

---

1. Steam the carrots and zucchini for 10-15 minutes until well cooked.
2. Meanwhile, add the oil to a wok over a medium-high heat.
3. Add the ground chicken and cook for 10 minutes or until browned.
4. Now add the grated carrots, zucchini, cooked noodles and allspice to the chicken and stir for 5 minutes.
5. Serve.

Per serving: Calories: 169; Fat: 6g (Saturated Fat: 4g); Carbohydrates: 10g; Fiber: 1g; Sugar: 1g; Sodium: 289mg; Protein: 18g

# TURKEY MEATBALLS & ZUCCHINI SPAGHETTI

**SERVES 4 / PREP TIME: 5 MINUTES / COOK TIME: 30 MINUTES**

These meatballs are flavorsome and tender - great for the stomach.

---

**8OZ LEAN GROUND TURKEY**

**1 TBSP FRESH PARSLEY, CHOPPED**

**1 EGG WHITE**

**1 TSP OLIVE OIL**

**2 CUPS ZUCCHINI, PEELED AND SPIRAL-IZED**

---

1. Mix the ground turkey with the parsley and egg white.
2. Use the palms of your hands to form 8 meatballs.
3. Heat the oil in a skillet over a medium-high heat and add the meatballs.
4. Brown each side, carefully turning with a cooking spoon.
5. Leave to cook through for 15-20 minutes.
6. When the meatballs are nearly done, place a pan of water (4 cups) over a high heat and bring to the boil.
7. Add the zucchini noodles for 7-8 minutes, drain and plunge into iced water.
8. Serve 2 meatballs over 1/4 of the zucchini and enjoy.

Per serving: Calories: 148; Fat: 8g (Saturated Fat: 2g); Carbohydrates: 4g; Fiber: 1g; Sugar: 2g; Sodium: 79mg; Protein: 16g

# SHRIMP PAELLA

**SERVES 4 / PREP TIME: 5 MINUTES / COOK TIME: 45 MINUTES**

A tasty Mediterranean inspired dish.

---

**1 TBSP OLIVE OIL**

**8OZ SHRIMP, PEELED & DE-VEINED**

**1/2 CUP CANNED MUSHROOMS**

**1/4 CUP CANNED PUMPKIN**

**1 CUP WHITE RICE, UNCOOKED**

**1 CUP LOW SODIUM CHICKEN STOCK**

**1 CUP WATER**

**2 TBSP FRESH CILANTRO, CHOPPED**

---

1. In a large pan or work, heat the oil over a medium-high heat.
2. Add the shrimp and cook until they turn pink.
3. Now add the mushrooms and canned pumpkin and sauté for a further 10-15 minutes.
4. Add the rice, water and stock to the pan, cover and simmer for 20-25 minutes or until the rice has cooked through and the stock has been absorbed into the rice.
5. Serve hot with freshly chopped cilantro.

Per serving: Calories: 144; Fat: 2g (Saturated Fat: 0g); Carbohydrates: 15g; Fiber: 1g; Sugar: 1g; Sodium: 406mg; Protein: 17g

# TILAPIA AND PAPAYA

**SERVES 4 / PREP TIME: 10 MINUTES / COOK TIME: 40 MINUTES**

An exotic blend of fish that works brilliantly with the sweet papaya.

---

**1/2 ACORN SQUASH, PEELED AND DICED**

**1 TBSP COCONUT OIL**

**4OZ TILAPIA FILLET, SKINLESS AND DE-BONED**

**1/4 CUP CANNED PAPAYA (SKINLESS)**

**1 TBSP FRESH CILANTRO, CHOPPED**

---

1. Bring a pan of water (6 cups) to the boil over a high heat.
2. Add the diced squash, reduce heat slightly and simmer for 30-40 minutes or until very soft.
3. Meanwhile, heat the coconut oil in a skillet over a medium heat.
4. Add the tilapia and cook for 10-15 minutes or until cooked through.
5. Remove fish and place to one side.
6. Use a knife and fork to shred the fish into small pieces.
7. Add the papaya to the skillet and heat through.
8. Serve the tilapia with the squash and the papaya and toss through to mix.
9. Garnish with fresh cilantro and sea salt to serve.

Per serving: Calories: 105; Fat: 4g (Saturated Fat: 3g); Carbohydrates: 13g; Fiber: 1.5g; Sugar: 0.5g; Sodium: 19.5mg; Protein: 5g

# POACHED COD & MINTED YELLOW SQUASH

**SERVES 4 / PREP TIME: 5 MINUTES / COOK TIME: 20 MINUTES**

Gentle on the stomach, this fish dish is also a home favorite.

---

**8OZ COD FILLET, DE-BONED AND SKINLESS**

**1 CUP SKIM MILK OR EQUIVALENT**

**1 TBSP PARSLEY**

**1 CUP YELLOW SQUASH, PEELED AND DICED**

**1 CUP COOKED WHITE RICE**

---

1. Check your fish for any remaining bones and remove with tweezers.
2. Add the milk and parsley to a pan over a medium-high heat and poach the cod in the milk for 20 minutes or until cooked through.
3. Meanwhile, steam the yellow squash over the same pan until very soft.
4. Use the back of a spoon to push the squash through a strainer.
5. Remove the cod and break up with a fork to check again for any bones (keep the milk in the pan).
6. Serve the cod, a helping of the parsley milk, and the squash purée over the rice.

Per serving: Calories: 128; Fat: 1g (Saturated Fat: 0g); Carbohydrates: 16g; Fiber: 1g; Sugar: 4g; Sodium: 61mg; Protein: 13g

# BAKED POTATO & TURKEY TOPPER

**SERVES 4 / PREP TIME: 5 MINUTES / COOK TIME: 40 MINUTES**

A healthy jacket potato lunch.

---

**2 LARGE BAKING POTATOES**

**1 TSP OLIVE OIL**

**7OZ LEAN GROUND TURKEY**

**2 SCALLIONS, CHOPPED**

**1 TBSP HOMEMADE TOMATO PASTE**

---

1. Preheat oven to 400°F/200 °C/Gas Mark 6.
2. Pierce the potato skins with a fork.
3. Add to the oven for 25-30 minutes or until cooked through.
4. Meanwhile, heat the oil in a skillet over a medium heat and add the ground turkey until browned.
5. Stir in the scallions and tomato paste and leave to simmer for 25-30 minutes or until cooked through.
6. Once potatoes are soft in the middle, slice in half and top with the turkey mixture and enjoy.
7. Please note: This recipe avoids the potato skins so please just eat the potato flesh from the inside!

Per serving: Calories: 169; Fat: 7g (Saturated Fat: 2g); Carbohydrates: 13g; Fiber: 1g; Sugar: 2g; Sodium: 51mg; Protein: 14g

# OVEN-BAKED COD WITH CRUSHED PETITE POTATOES

**SERVES 4 / PREP TIME: 5 MINUTES / COOK TIME: 20 MINUTES**

A light and refreshing entrée.

---

**8OZ COD FILLET, DE-BONED AND SKINLESS**

**12 PETITE POTATOES (OR 4 SMALL WHITE POTATOES), PEELED**

**1 TBSP DILL, FRESHLY CHOPPED**

**1 TSP OLIVE OIL**

---

1. Preheat oven to 375°F/190 °C/Gas Mark 5.
2. Wrap cod in parchment paper.
3. Bake in the oven for 10-15 minutes or until cooked through.
4. Meanwhile, boil a pot of water over a high heat and add the potatoes.
5. Leave to boil for 10-15 minutes or until soft.
6. Drain potatoes and crush with a fork.
7. Mix the dill and olive oil together and drizzle over the cod and potatoes. Season with black pepper to taste.

Per serving: Calories: 135; Fat: 2g (Saturated Fat: 0g); Carbohydrates: 19g; Fiber: 2g; Sugar: 1g; Sodium: 261mg; Protein: 11g

# HERBY HEALTHY FISH CAKES

**SERVES 4 / PREP TIME: 5 MINUTES / COOK TIME: 40 MINUTES**

Deliciously satisfying!

---

1 LARGE WHITE POTATO, PEELED AND CHOPPED

1/2 CUP SKIM MILK OR EQUIVALENT

8 OZ COD FILLETS (OR OTHER WHITE FISH), DE-BONED AND SKINLESS

1 CUP WATER

2 SCALLION STEMS, CHOPPED

1 TSP DRIED DILL, CHOPPED

1 TSP DRIED PARSLEY, CHOPPED

1 EGG WHITE

1 TSP OLIVE OIL

---

1. Boil the potato in a pot of water over a high heat for 20 minutes or until very soft and fluffy.
2. Meanwhile, bring the milk to almost boiling point in a separate pan over a high heat.
3. Add the cod and water to the pan of milk and lower the heat slightly.
4. Allow to simmer for 25 minutes or until fish is thoroughly cooked through.
5. Drain and flake with a knife and fork.
6. Drain the potato and mash until smooth.
7. Mix in the flaked fish, scallions, herbs and then add the egg white to bind.
8. Using your hands, shape into 4 patties.
9. Heat the oil in a skillet over a medium-high heat and cook the fish cakes for 2 minutes on each side to brown and crispy.

Per serving: Calories: 137; Fat: 2g (Saturated Fat: 0g); Carbohydrates: 17g; Fiber: 2g; Sugar: 2g; Sodium: 257mg; Protein: 13g

# CHICKEN WITH SPINACH & NUTMEG STUFFING

**SERVES 4 / PREP TIME: 10 MINUTES / COOK TIME: 25 MINUTES**

Juicy chicken with iron-rich stuffing.

---

| | |
|---|---|
| **2X 4OZ CHICKEN BREASTS, SKINLESS** | **1 TSP NUTMEG, GROUND** |
| **1 TSP UNSALTED BUTTER** | **1 SALTINE CRACKER, CRUSHED** |
| **1 CUP BABY SPINACH** | **2 SHEETS OF PLASTIC WRAP** |

---

1. Preheat oven to 375°F/190 °C/Gas Mark 5.
2. Butterfly each chicken breast and place flat on the left edge of the plastic wrap.
3. Fold the right edge of the plastic wrap over each chicken breast and use a rolling pin or meat pounder to flatten the chicken to 1/2 cm thick.
4. Heat the butter in a small pan over a medium heat and add the spinach and nutmeg for 3-4 minutes or until the spinach has melted.
5. Remove from the heat and add the crushed crackers - mix well.
6. Unfold the plastic wrap from the chicken and spread the stuffing over the chicken breasts.
7. Now pick up the corners of the plastic wrap closest to you and carefully roll the chicken breast away from you.
8. Add the chicken rolls to an oven dish filled with hot water.
9. Place in the oven for 25-20 minutes or until thoroughly cooked through.
10. Cut each roll in half and serve hot with your choice of side.

Per serving: Calories: 115; Fat: 4g (Saturated Fat: 1g); Carbohydrates: 3g; Fiber: 1g; Sugar: 0g; Sodium: 315mg; Protein: 18g

# MUSSEL LINGUINE

**SERVES 4 / PREP TIME: 5 MINUTES / COOK TIME: 15 MINUTES**

A fresh seafood pasta dish.

---

**1 CUP WHITE LINGUINE (OR ANY PASTA OF YOUR CHOICE)**

**1 CUP LOW SODIUM VEGETABLE (OR FISH) STOCK**

**8OZ MUSSELS (WITHOUT SHELLS)**

**1 TBSP FRESH PARSLEY, CHOPPED**

**1 TBSP OLIVE OIL**

---

1. Bring a pot of water (3 cups) to the boil over a high heat.
2. Add the pasta, lower the heat, and allow to simmer for 10-15 minutes or according to package directions.
3. In a separate pan, add the stock and mussels and cook over a medium heat until fish turns opaque (10-15 minutes or according to package directions).
4. Drain the pasta and add to the mussels.
5. Sprinkle with parsley and drizzle with olive oil to serve.

Per serving: Calories: 174; Fat: 5g (Saturated Fat: 1g); Carbohydrates: 20g; Fiber: 1g; Sugar: 1g; Sodium: 349mg; Protein: 11g

# SHRIMP SPAGHETTI

**SERVES 2 / PREP TIME: 5 MINUTES / COOK TIME: 20 MINUTES**

A taste of the Mediterranean!

---

1/2 CUP (4OZ) SPAGHETTI NOODLES

1 TSP OLIVE OIL

4OZ SHRIMP

1 TBSP LOW SODIUM TOMATO PASTE

1/4 CUP HOMEMADE FISH/VEGETABLE STOCK

1 TBSP FRESH CILANTRO, CHOPPED

---

1. Bring a pot of water to the boil over a high heat.
2. Add the pasta, lower the heat, and allow to simmer for 10-15 minutes or according to package directions.
3. In a separate skillet, add the olive oil and sauté the shrimp over a medium heat for 10 minutes or until shrimp turns opaque.
4. Stir in the tomato paste and stock and allow to simmer for a further 10 minutes.
5. Drain the pasta and add to the skillet with the shrimps.
6. Toss to mix.
7. Sprinkle with cilantro to serve.

Per serving: Calories: 287; Fat: 4g (Saturated Fat: 1g); Carbohydrates: 43g; Fiber: 3g; Sugar: 2g; Sodium: 565mg; Protein: 18g; Potassium: 207mg

# GINGERED CLAM NOODLES

**SERVES 2  /  PREP TIME: 5 MINUTES /  COOK TIME: 25 MINUTES**

A hint of the orient.

| | |
|---|---|
| 1/2 CUP EGG NOODLES | 4OZ CLAMS |
| 1 TSP COCONUT OIL | 1 TSP GINGER PASTE |
| 1/2 CUP MUSHROOMS | 1 TBSP CHINESE FLAT LEAF PARSLEY |

1. Cook the egg noodles in a pan of boiling water (1 cup) for 10-15 minutes or according to package directions.
2. Meanwhile, heat the oil in a skillet over a medium-high heat and add the mushrooms.
3. Sauté for 10 minutes until thoroughly cooked through.
4. Now add the clams, cook for 5-10 minutes or until cooked through.
5. Now add the ginger paste and stir.
6. Drain the noodles and top with the shrimp and mushrooms.
7. Sprinkle over the Chinese flat-leaf parsley and serve.

Per serving: Calories: 116; Fat: 4g (Saturated Fat: 2g); Carbohydrates: 16g; Fiber: 1g; Sugar: 1g; Sodium: 90mg; Protein: 5g; Potassium: 155mg

# GINGER & SCALLION SHRIMP

**SERVES 4 / PREP TIME: 5 MINUTES / COOK TIME: 15 MINUTES**

Aromatic and flavorsome.

---

| | |
|---|---|
| **1 CUP EGG NOODLES** | **1 TSP GINGER, GRATED** |
| **1 TSP COCONUT OIL** | **2 SCALLIONS STEMS, CHOPPED** |
| **8OZ SHRIMP** | |

---

1. Cook the egg noodles according to package directions.
2. Heat the oil in a skillet over a high heat and add the shrimp for 10 minutes or until pink.
3. Now add the grated ginger and chopped scallions and stir for a few minutes.
4. Top the noodles with the shrimp.
5. Serve.

Per serving: Calories: 101; Fat: 2g (Saturated Fat: 1g); Carbohydrates: 8g; Fiber: 1g; Sugar: 0g; Sodium: 469mg; Protein: 11g

# CHICKEN SATAY SKEWERS WITH WHITE RICE

**SERVES 4 / PREP TIME: 10 MINUTES / COOK TIME: 30 MINUTES**

Nutty chicken delight.

---

1 TBSP ALMOND BUTTER

1 TBSP TOMATO PASTE

1 TBSP WATER

8OZ CHICKEN BREAST, SKINLESS

1 CUP WHITE RICE

4 SMALL METAL SKEWERS

---

1. Mix the almond butter with the tomato paste and water to make your satay sauce.
2. Cut your chicken into small cubes and marinate in the satay sauce for as long as possible.
3. Preheat broiler to a medium-high heat.
4. Skewer the marinated chicken and place on a baking tray.
5. Then use the remaining marinade to brush over the skewers.
6. Place under the broiler for 25-30 minutes or until chicken is thoroughly cooked through.
7. Meanwhile, add the rice to a pan of cold water (2 cups) and bring to the boil over a high heat.
8. Lower the heat and simmer for 20 minutes or until most of the water is absorbed.
9. Drain and cover to steam.
10. Once chicken is done, remove from broiler and serve with a helping of white rice.

Per serving: Calories: 168; Fat: 4g (Saturated Fat: 1g); Carbohydrates: 13g; Fiber: 1g; Sugar: 1g; Sodium: 268mg; Protein: 19g

# SEA BASS WITH BASIL PESTO MASH

**SERVES 4 / PREP TIME: 10 MINUTES / COOK TIME: 35 MINUTES**

The herby mash tastes great with this meaty white fish.

---

**1 WHITE POTATO, PEELED AND DICED**

**1 TBSP OLIVE OIL**

**1/4 CUP FRESH BASIL, FINELY CHOPPED**

**1 TBSP UNSALTED BUTTER**

**4OZ SEA BASS FILLET, SKINLESS**

---

1. Place the potato and 1 tbsp olive oil in a microwavable zip lock bag.
2. Place this into the microwave for 20 minutes (alternatively, boil in a pot for 25 minutes).
3. Meanwhile, heat 1 tbsp olive oil in a skillet over a medium-high heat and cook the sea bass fillet for 6 minutes.
4. Turn and cook the over side for 4 minutes (ensure fish is thoroughly cooked through).
5. Remove from the heat and place to one side.
6. Once cooked, remove the potato from the microwave and very carefully unzip the bag (it will be steaming hot).
7. Pop the potato into a large bowl and mash with a potato masher.
8. Mix in the chopped basil and butter and allow to melt.
9. Gently flake the sea bass fillet and serve on top of the basil mash.

Hint: Use olive oil instead of butter if lactose intolerant.

Per serving: Calories: 228; Fat: 13g (Saturated Fat: 5g); Carbohydrates: 17g; Fiber: 2g; Sugar: 1g; Sodium: 237mg; Protein: 11g; Potassium: 395mg

# CHICKEN AND ACORN SQUASH

**SERVES 4  /  PREP TIME: 10 MINUTES  /  COOK TIME: 30 MINUTES**

A tasty, healthy chicken dish - perfect for the fall.

1 CUP ACORN SQUASH, PEELED AND CUBED

2 CUPS WATER

8OZ CHICKEN BREAST, SKINLESS

1 TSP OLIVE OIL

1 CUP SPINACH

1 TBSP DRIED THYME

1. Add the cubed squash to a pan with the water.
2. Bring to the boil.
3. Allow to boil for 20-25 minutes or until soft.
4. Meanwhile, chop the chicken into small pieces.
5. Heat the olive oil in a skillet over a medium-high heat and add the chicken for 25-30 minutes or until cooked through.
6. Add the spinach to the skillet in the last 10 minutes and season with the thyme.
7. Drain the squash.
8. Serve the chicken and spinach on a bed of squash.
9. Enjoy!

Per serving: Calories: 126; Fat: 3g (Saturated Fat: 1g); Carbohydrates: 6g; Fiber: 2g; Sugar: 0g; Sodium: 309mg; Protein: 19g

# TURKEY BREAST & SCALLION SOUP

**SERVES 4  /  PREP TIME: 10 MINUTES  /  COOK TIME: 30 MINUTES**

A hearty Winter dish.

---

1 TSP OLIVE OIL

1/2 CUP CARROT, PEELED AND CHOPPED

1/4 CUP SCALLIONS, CHOPPED

7OZ LEAN TURKEY BREASTS, SLICED

1 CUP LOW SODIUM CHICKEN STOCK

2 CUPS WATER

1 BAY LEAF

1 LARGE WHITE POTATO, PEELED AND CHOPPED

1 TSP DRIED THYME

1 TSP DRIED ROSEMARY

---

1. Heat the oil in a large pot over a medium-high heat.
2. Add the carrots and scallions to the pot for 5 minutes.
3. Add the turkey and brown for 5 minutes.
4. Now add the stock and the rest of the ingredients before lowering the heat, covering and simmering for 20 minutes.
5. Serve piping hot in soup bowls

Per serving: Calories: 136; Fat: 1g (Saturated Fat: 0g); Carbohydrates: 18g; Fiber: 2g; Sugar: 2g; Sodium: 233mg; Protein: 14g

# TURKEY BOLOGNESE

**SERVES 6 /   PREP TIME: 10 MINUTES  / COOK TIME: 30 MINUTES**

Leaner than the traditional beef version - this tastes delicious. It is slightly higher in calories than the other recipes in this cookbook so remember to keep track of all your

1 TSP OLIVE OIL

9OZ LEAN GROUND TURKEY

1/4 CUP MUSHROOMS, SLICED

1/4 CUP CARROTS, PEELED AND SLICED

2 SCALLION STEMS, CHOPPED

1 TSP THYME

1/4 CUP LOW SODIUM TOMATO PASTE

1/2 CUP LOW SODIUM CHICKEN STOCK

10 OZ SPAGHETTI (OR GLUTEN-FREE EQUIVALENT)

1. Heat the oil in a skillet over a medium-high heat.
2. Add the ground turkey and stir to brown for 5 minutes.
3. Now add the vegetables and stir in for 5 minutes.
4. Add the tomato paste, thyme and stock.
5. Lower the heat and simmer for 20 minutes or until turkey is thoroughly cooked through.
6. Meanwhile, add a pot of water (4 cups) to the stove and bring to the boil.
7. Now add the spaghetti and simmer for 20 minutes or according to package directions.
8. Drain and serve with the turkey bolognese on top!

Per serving: Calories: 272; Fat: 7g (Saturated Fat: 2g); Carbohydrates: 35g; Fiber: 2g; Sugar: 1g; Sodium: 46mg; Protein: 18g

# TOMATO & COD STEW

**SERVES 4 / PREP TIME: 10 MINUTES / COOK TIME: 30 MINUTES**

Oven-baking keeps this cod soft and the flavor is amazing!

---

8OZ COD FILLETS, SKINLESS AND DE-BONED

1/4 CUP LOW SODIUM TOMATO PASTE

1/2 CUP LOW SODIUM VEGETABLE STOCK

1/2 CUP ZUCCHINI, PEELED AND CHOPPED

1/2 CUP CANNED PUMPKIN (SKINLESS)

1/2 CUP SPINACH

1 BAY LEAF

1 TBSP FRESH PARSLEY

1 TSP CILANTRO

---

1. Preheat oven to 375°F/190 °C/Gas Mark 5.
2. Into a lined baking dish, add all of the ingredients.
3. Cover and bake in the oven for 25-30 minutes or until fish is cooked through.
4. Serve with white rice if desired.

Per serving: Calories: 81; Fat: 1g (Saturated Fat: 0g); Carbohydrates: 8g; Fiber: 2g; Sugar: 4g; Sodium: 201mg; Protein: 12g

# WINTER-SPICED CHICKEN & YAMS

**SERVES 4 / PREP TIME: 10 MINUTES / COOK TIME: 45 MINUTES**

Succulent and filling!

---

| | |
|---|---|
| **8OZ CHICKEN BREAST, SKINLESS** | **1 CINNAMON STICK** |
| **2 TSP OLIVE OIL** | **1 TSP NUTMEG** |
| **1/2 CUP LOW SODIUM CHICKEN STOCK** | **1 TSP ALLSPICE** |
| **1 TSP GROUND GINGER** | |
| **1 YAM, PEELED AND CUBED** | |

---

1. Slice the chicken breasts.
2. Heat the oil in a large pot over a medium-high heat.
3. Add the chicken and brown each side for 5 minutes total.
4. Now add the rest of the ingredients.
5. Cover the pot, reduce the heat, and allow to simmer for 30-40 minutes or until chicken and yams are thoroughly cooked through.
6. Remove the cinnamon stick before serving.

Per serving: Calories: 139; Fat: 4g (Saturated Fat: 1g); Carbohydrates: 8g; Fiber: 1g; Sugar: 0g; Sodium: 296mg; Protein: 18g

# CHICKEN WITH BASIL, MOZZARELLA & TOMATO SAUCE

**SERVES 4 / PREP TIME: 10 MINUTES / COOK TIME: 40 MINUTES**

A scrumptious Italian-influenced chicken dish.

---

**2X 4OZ CHICKEN BREASTS, SKINLESS**

**1/4 CUP LOW-FAT MOZZARELLA**

**2 TBSP BASIL, FRESHLY CHOPPED**

**1 CUP WHITE RICE**

**1/4 CUP HOMEMADE TOMATO SAUCE**

---

1. Preheat the oven to 350°f/170°c/Gas Mark 4.
2. Using a sharp knife, make a slice through the center of the chicken (enough to create a pocket but not all the way through).
3. Stuff with the mozzarella and basil.
4. Wrap in foil and place in the oven for 30-35 minutes or until chicken is thoroughly cooked through.
5. Meanwhile, add the rice to a pot of water (2 cups) on a high heat.
6. Bring to the boil and then lower the heat and simmer for 20 minutes.
7. Once the rice has soaked up most of the water, drain and cover to steam.
8. 5 minutes before the chicken is done unwrap and check it is cooked through. Remove the foil and pour the tomato sauce over the chicken.
9. Continue to cook uncovered for 10 minutes or until heated through.
10. Serve the rice with 1/2 chicken breast each and a helping of tomato sauce.


Per serving: Calories: 158; Fat: 2g (Saturated Fat: 0g); Carbohydrates: 6g; Fiber: 13g; Sugar: 1g; Sodium: 334mg; Protein: 20g

# SCALLOPS WITH APPLE & SCALLIONS

**SERVES 4 / PREP TIME: 5 MINUTES / COOK TIME: 10 MINUTES**

A little bit of luxury!

---

**1 TBSP OLIVE OIL**

**12 SCALLOPS**

**1/4 CUP APPLESAUCE**

**2 SCALLION STEMS, FINELY CHOPPED**

---

1. Heat the olive oil in a skillet over a medium-high heat.
2. Add the scallops for 1-2 minutes on each side or until scallops are opaque.
3. Now lower the heat add the scallions for 1 minute.
4. Now add the apple sauce for 1-2 minutes.
5. The apple sauce will add a lovely sticky glaze to the scallops and scallions - don't let the scallions brown!
6. Serve immediately and enjoy - check the scallops are cooked through (they should be opaque and firm yet still soft to touch).

Per serving: Calories: 57; Fat: 0g (Saturated Fat: 0g); Carbohydrates: 5g; Fiber: 0g; Sugar: 3g; Sodium: 204mg; Protein: 8g

# SMOKED HALIBUT KEDGEREE

**SERVES 4 / PREP TIME: 5 MINUTES / COOK TIME: 30 MINUTES**

Using alternative ingredients, this is still a winner!

---

| | |
|---|---|
| 1 TSP UNSALTED BUTTER/OLIVE OIL | 1 TSP ALLSPICE |
| 8OZ SMOKED HALIBUT, SKINLESS AND DE-BONED | 1 TSP PARSLEY, CHOPPED |
| | 1/2 CUP LOW SODIUM VEG STOCK |
| 1 CUP WHITE RICE | 1 1/2 CUPS WATER |
| 1/2 CUP SPINACH | 1 TBSP FAT FREE GREEK YOGURT |

---

1. Heat the butter/oil in a large pot over a medium-high heat.
2. Add the smoked haddock and cook for 5 minutes.
3. Now add the rest of the ingredients (apart from the yogurt), cover and simmer for 25-30 minutes.
4. Keep an eye on the pot and stir throughout to ensure the ingredients don't burn - add a little extra water if necessary.
5. Most of the stock should be absorbed once cooked.
6. Stir in the Greek yogurt and serve right away.

Per serving: Calories: 198; Fat: 3g (Saturated Fat: 1g); Carbohydrates: 13g; Fiber: 1g; Sugar: 0g; Sodium: 385mg; Protein: 28g

# POLLOCK EN PAPILLOTE

SERVES 2 / PREP TIME: 5 MINUTES / COOK TIME: 25 MINUTES

Flaky white fish with potatoes - a taste of home!

---

**1 SMALL WHITE POTATO, PEELED AND CUBED**

**1 SHEET PARCHMENT PAPER**

**4OZ POLLOCK FILLET, SKINLESS AND DE-BONED (OR OTHER WHITE FISH OF CHOICE)**

**1 TSP OLIVE OIL**

**1 TBSP FRESH PARSLEY**

---

1. Preheat the oven to 190°C/375°F/Gas Mark 5.
2. Bring a small pot of water to the boil over a high heat.
3. Add the cubed potato and lower the heat slightly.
4. Cook for 15-20 minutes or until very soft.
5. Meanwhile, lay out the parchment paper on an oven tray.
6. Place the pollock fillet onto the paper and drizzle over the olive oil.
7. Add the parsley.
8. Fold the paper over and lightly scrunch the edges together to make a loose parcel.
9. Add to the oven for 15-18 minutes or until fish is thoroughly cooked through and flakes easily.
10. Now drain the potato, slice in half, season to taste and serve on the side of half of the fish.
11. Enjoy!

Per serving: Calories: 119; Fat: 3g (Saturated Fat: 0g); Carbohydrates: 13g; Fiber: 1g; Sugar: 1g; Sodium: 186mg; Protein: 11g

# FRAGRANT CHICKEN CURRY

**SERVES 2 / PREP TIME: 5 MINUTES / COOK TIME: 30 MINUTES**

A mild yet fragrant chicken curry.

---

4OZ CHICKEN BREAST, BONELESS & SKINLESS

1/2 TBSP GARLIC INFUSED OIL

1 TSP SWEET CURRY POWDER

1 TBSP TOMATO PASTE

1 BAY LEAF

1 CINNAMON STICK

1/2 CUP LOW SODIUM CHICKEN STOCK

1 CUP WATER

1 TBSP FRESH CILANTRO, CHOPPED

---

1. Dice the chicken into bite-size cubes.
2. Heat a large wok or pot over a medium heat.
3. Add the oil to melt.
4. Sauté chicken pieces until golden brown.
5. Now add the curry powder, tomato paste, bay leaf, cinnamon stick, water and chicken stock.
6. Simmer for 20 minutes.
7. Ensure the chicken is thoroughly cooked through before serving with the fresh cilantro scattered over the top.
8. Enjoy with white rice or bread to mop up the flavors.

Per serving: Calories: 139; Fat: 6g (Saturated Fat: 1g); Carbohydrates: 3g; Fiber: 1g; Sugar: 1.g; Sodium: 299mg; Protein: 19g

# CREAMY CHICKEN & MUSHROOM SOUP

**SERVES 2 / PREP TIME: 5 MINUTES / COOK TIME: 15 MINUTES**

A winter warmer.

---

| | |
|---|---|
| 4OZ ROASTED AND SKINLESS CHICKEN BREAST | 1 TSP DRIED DILL |
| 1/2 CUP LOW-SODIUM CHICKEN STOCK | 1 TSP DRIED THYME |
| 1 CUP WATER | 1 TSP BLACK PEPPER |
| 1/4 CUP COOKED EGG NOODLES | 1/4 CUP SKIM MILK (OR DAIRY-FREE EQUIVALENT) |
| 1 CUP MUSHROOMS, COOKED | |

---

1. Use leftover chicken or alternatively, roast the chicken in foil in the oven for 25-30 minutes or until thoroughly cooked through prior to preparing the soup. (Heat oven to 190°C/375°F/Gas Mark 5 to cook).
2. Slice the chicken.
3. Now add the stock and water to a pot over a high heat and bring to the boil.
4. Add the chicken, noodles, mushrooms, herbs and pepper.
5. Turn down the heat slightly, stir in the milk, and allow to simmer for 10 minutes.
6. Remove from the heat and allow to cool slightly.
7. Blend in food processor for a smooth, creamy soup.

Hint: No need to blend if you can handle solid foods.

Per serving: Calories: 133; Fat: 5.5g (Saturated Fat: 0g); Carbohydrates: 13g; Fiber: 2g; Sugar: 3g; Sodium: 133.5mg; Protein: 21.5g

# PARSLEY BUTTER HADDOCK

**SERVES 2 / PREP TIME: 5 MINUTES / COOK TIME: 30 MINUTES**

Buttery poached fish with crushed new potatoes.

---

**1/2 CUP PEELED PETITE POTATOES**

**4OZ HADDOCK FILLET, DE-BONED AND SKINLESS (OR OTHER WHITE FISH)**

**2 CUPS SKIM MILK (OR DAIRY-FREE)**

**1 TBSP UNSALTED BUTTER (USE OLIVE OIL IF LACTOSE INTOLERANT)**

**1/4 CUP FRESH PARSLEY, CHOPPED**

---

1. Bring a pot of water to the boil and add the peeled baby potatoes.
2. Lower the heat slightly and allow to simmer for 15-20 minutes.
3. Meanwhile, add the milk to a separate pot over a medium-high heat.
4. Add the haddock and allow to poach in the milk for 15-20 minutes or until thoroughly cooked through.
5. Drain potatoes and haddock (reserve 1 tbsp of the milk).
6. Use a fork to crush the potatoes with the reserved milk.
7. Heat the butter in a skillet over a medium heat.
8. Add the chopped parsley to the skillet once melted.
9. Plate up the potatoes and haddock and drizzle over the delicious parsley butter.
10. Season with pepper to taste.
11. Enjoy!

Per serving: Calories: 150; Fat: 6g (Saturated Fat: 4g); Carbohydrates: 12g; Fiber: 1g; Sugar: 1g; Sodium: 179mg; Protein: 11g; Potassium: 345mg

# CHICKEN WITH CARROT & SQUASH PURÉE

**SERVES 2 / PREP TIME: 5 MINUTES / COOK TIME: 30 MINUTES**

Lightly spiced chicken with a sweet side.

---

**1/4 CUP ACORN SQUASH PEELED AND CHOPPED**

**1 TSP GROUND NUTMEG**

**1/2 TSP BLACK PEPPER**

**1 SMALL CARROT, PEELED AND CHOPPED**

**1/2 TBSP OLIVE OIL**

**4OZ CHICKEN BREASTS, SKINLESS AND SLICED**

**1/2 TSP DRIED ROSEMARY**

---

1. Bring a pot of water to the boil and add the squash, nutmeg and black pepper.
2. Cook for 25-30 minutes or until very soft.
3. Add the carrots for the last 20 minutes.
4. Meanwhile, heat the oil in a skillet over a medium-high heat.
5. Add the sliced chicken and stir to brown.
6. Sprinkle over the rosemary and continue to sauté for 20 minutes.
7. Check chicken is thoroughly cooked through - it should not be pink in the middle.
8. Drain vegetables and allow to cool slightly.
9. Blend in a food processor until smooth.
10. Serve sliced chicken on a helping of purée and enjoy.

Per serving: Calories: 74; Fat: 4g (Saturated Fat: 1); Carbohydrates: 4g; Fiber: 1g; Sugar: 1g; Sodium: 83mg; Protein: 5g; Potassium: 173mg

# VEGETARIAN ENTRÉES

# MIGHTY RICE SALAD

**SERVES 4 / PREP TIME: 10 MINUTES / COOK TIME: 30 MINUTES**

A wholesome, tasty and low-fat salad.

---

**1 CUP YELLOW SQUASH, PEELED AND DICED**

**1 CUP WHITE RICE**

**1 CUP SPINACH**

**1 TBSP CILANTRO, FRESHLY CHOPPED**

**1 TSP OLIVE OIL**

---

1. Steam the squash over boiling water for 30 minutes or until soft.
2. Meanwhile, add the rice to a pan of cold water (2 cups) and bring to the boil.
3. Lower the heat and simmer for 20 minutes.
4. Wash the spinach and steam with the squash for the last 10 minutes.
5. Once the rice has soaked up most of the water and the squash is very soft, drain and mix all of the ingredients together to form your salad.
6. Whisk olive oil with fresh cilantro and drizzle over the rice to serve.

Per serving: Calories: 102; Fat: 2g (Saturated Fat: 0g); Carbohydrates: 15g; Fiber: 2g; Sugar: 2g; Sodium: 33mg; Protein: 3g

# SUMMER SQUASH STEW & BAKED EGGS

**SERVES 4 / PREP TIME: 10 MINUTES / COOK TIME: 50 MINUTES**

A rustic dish.

---

1 SUMMER SQUASH, HALVED

1 TBSP OLIVE OIL

1 ZUCCHINI, CUBED, SEEDS REMOVED
FROM CENTRE

1 TSP THYME

1/2 CUP CANNED TOMATOES (SKINLESS)

1/2 CUP 'HOMEMADE VEG STOCK'

4 EGGS

1 TBSP CILANTRO, FRESHLY CHOPPED

---

1. Preheat oven to 300°F/150 °C/Gas Mark 2.
2. Place the summer squash flesh side down in a shallow oven dish with 1 cup water.
3. Bake for 30-40 minutes or until squash very soft.
4. Meanwhile, heat the oil in a pot over a medium-high heat and add the zucchini, thyme, tomatoes and stock.
5. Lower the heat, cover and simmer until the squash is ready.
6. Once the squash is cooked through, remove and allow to cool; then use a spoon to scoop out the flesh from the inside.
7. Add the flesh to the tomato stew on the stove and stir through.
8. Turn the oven off and the broiler on to high.
9. Add the stew to the oven dish that you cooked the squash in and crack the eggs on the top.
10. Place under the broiler for 5-6 minutes or until eggs are cooked through.
11. Sprinkle with cilantro to serve.

Per serving: Calories: 137; Fat: 9g (Saturated Fat: 2g); Carbohydrates: 7g; Fiber: 1g; Sugar: 2g; Sodium: 74mg; Protein: 8g

# SILKEN TOFU NOODLES

SERVES 4  /  PREP TIME: 5 MINUTES  /  COOK TIME: 15 MINUTES

A protein and vitamin packed noodle dish.

---

1 TBSP COCONUT OIL

1 CUP SILKEN TOFU

4 SCALLIONS, FINELY CHOPPED

1 CARROT, PEELED AND GRATED

1/2 CUP CHINESE MUSHROOMS, SOAKED

1 TSP GINGER, GRATED

1 CUP EGG NOODLES, COOKED

---

1. Heat the coconut oil in a wok or non-stick skillet on a high heat.
2. Add the tofu and brown for 5-10 minutes.
3. Now throw in the rest of the ingredients for 10-15 minutes or until all thoroughly cooked through.
4. Toss and serve.

Per serving: Calories: 146; Fat: 6g (Saturated Fat: 3g); Carbohydrates: 16g; Fiber: 2g; Sugar: 2g; Sodium: 24mg; Protein: 9g

# SPINACH & SQUASH LASAGNA

**SERVES 6 / PREP TIME: 10 MINUTES / COOK TIME: 45 MINUTES**

Bubbling and golden, this melts in your mouth!

**FOR THE WHITE SAUCE:**

**1 TBSP UNSALTED BUTTER**

**1/8 CUP ALMOND MEAL**

**1 CUP SKIM MILK OR EQUIVALENT**

**1 ACORN SQUASH, PEELED AND THINLY SLICED**

**2 CUPS BABY SPINACH**

1. Preheat the oven to 350°f/170°c/Gas Mark 4.
2. Heat the butter in a small pan over a low-medium heat.
3. Tilt the pan towards you so that the butter melts only on the near side of the pan as much as possible.
4. Add the almond meal to the far side of the pan and slowly mix this into the melted butter using a wooden spoon.
5. Once a paste is formed, add the milk slowly and stir continuously for approximately 10-15 minutes or until the lumps disappear (don't worry, they will!)
6. Now, line a lasagna dish with 1/2 squash slices.
7. Create a layer with 1/3 baby spinach.
8. Top with 1/3 white sauce.
9. Repeat 2 more layers with the rest of the ingredients and place in the oven for 30 minutes or until golden and bubbling.
10. Enjoy!

Per serving: Calories: 54; Fat: 3g (Saturated Fat: 1g); Carbohydrates: 4g; Fiber: 1g; Sugar: 2g; Sodium: 28mg; Protein: 3g

# SPINACH FLORENTINES

**SERVES 4 / PREP TIME: 10 MINUTES / COOK TIME: 30 MINUTES**

Amazing bite-size meals.

---

**2 CUPS BABY SPINACH**

**1 SWEET POTATO, PEELED AND CUBED**

**1 TBSP OLIVE OIL**

**2 SCALLION STEMS, CHOPPED**

---

1. Place the spinach, sweet potato and olive oil in a microwavable zip lock bag.
2. Place this into the microwave for 20 minutes. Alternatively, boil in a pot of water for 25 minutes.
3. Remove the sweet potato from the microwave and very carefully unzip the bag (it will be steaming hot).
4. Pop the sweet potato and spinach mixture into a large bowl and mash with a fork or potato masher.
5. Stir in the scallions.
6. Use wet hands to form palm size sweet potato 'cakes'.
7. Heat the oil in a skillet over a medium-high heat.
8. Add the florentines to the skillet and cook for 4 minutes on each side or until golden and slightly crispy.
9. Enjoy!

Per serving: Calories: 79; Fat: 4g (Saturated Fat: 0g); Carbohydrates: 10g; Fiber: 1g; Sugar: 4g; Sodium: 27mg; Protein: 1g

# PUMPKIN POTATO SALAD

**SERVES 4 / PREP TIME: 5 MINUTES / COOK TIME: 15 MINUTES**

Delicious!

---

**3 SMALL WHITE POTATOES, PEELED AND QUARTERED**

**1/2 CUP CANNED PUMPKIN**

**1 TBSP CHIVES, FRESHLY CHOPPED**

**1 TBSP DRIED DILL**

**1 TSP OLIVE OIL**

---

1. Add the potatoes to a pot of water and bring to the boil over a high heat.
2. Lower the heat slightly and simmer for 15 minutes or until the potatoes are very soft.
3. Meanwhile cook canned pumpkin according to package directions.
4. Drain potatoes.
5. Add to a large salad bowl along with the rest of the ingredients.
6. Toss to coat before serving.

Per serving: Calories: 57; Fat: 1g (Saturated Fat: 0g); Carbohydrates: 11g; Fiber: 2g; Sugar: 1g; Sodium: 50mg; Protein: 1g

# SQUASH STUFFED WITH COTTAGE CHEESE

**SERVES 8 / PREP TIME: 10 MINUTES / COOK TIME: 50 MINUTES**

A great sharing dish!

---

**1 CUP LOW-FAT COTTAGE CHEESE**

**1/2 CUP CANNED PINEAPPLE**

**1 ACORN SQUASH**

**3 SPRIGS THYME**

---

1. Preheat the oven to 375°f/190°c/Gas Mark 5.
2. Mix the cottage cheese and pineapple.
3. Slice a small slice from the bottom of the squash so that it can stand upright.
4. Cut a lid from the top of the squash.
5. Use a sharp knife to cut into the center of the squash and then a spoon to scrape out the seeds.
6. Place on a baking tray in the oven for 40 minutes or until the squash is very soft.
7. Stuff with the cottage cheese and pineapple and stick the thyme sprigs in the top for a further 10 minutes or until golden and bubbly.
8. Dig in!

Per serving: Calories: 53; Fat: 1g (Saturated Fat: 0g); Carbohydrates: 8g; Fiber: 1g; Sugar: 3g; Sodium: 95mg; Protein: 4g

# BAKED BEETS & RICOTTA PITA BREADS

**SERVES 2 / PREP TIME: 5 MINUTES / COOK TIME: 50 MINUTES**

Deliciously sweet and savory mini pizzas.

---

| | |
|---|---|
| **1 TSP UNSALTED BUTTER** | **A PINCH SEA SALT** |
| **1 WHOLE BEET, SCRUBBED AND SLICED** | **2 MEDIUM WHITE PITA BREADS** |
| **1 TSP STEVIA POWDER** | **1/2 CUP LOW-FAT RICOTTA** |

---

1. Preheat the oven to 375°f/190°c/Gas Mark 5.
2. Heat the butter in a skillet over a medium heat.
3. Add the beet, stevia and sea salt.
4. Transfer to a baking tray, cover with foil and roast in the oven for 30-40 minutes.
5. When the beets are soft, remove.
6. Turn the broiler on to a medium heat.
7. Slice the pita breads in half and place on a baking dish for 4-5 minutes.
8. Remove and spread the ricotta on top, then add the beets.
9. Place under the broiler for a few minutes until the ricotta starts to bubble.
10. Remove and enjoy!

Per serving: Calories: 238; Fat: 7g (Saturated Fat: 4g); Carbohydrates: 32g; Fiber: 1g; Sugar: 3g; Sodium: 338mg; Protein: 12g

# MUSHROOM RISOTTO

**SERVES 4 / PREP TIME: 5 MINUTES / COOK TIME: 40 MINUTES**

Woody textured risotto.

---

**1 TBSP OLIVE OIL**

**1/4 CUP SCALLIONS, CHOPPED**

**2 CUPS MUSHROOMS, SLICED**

**2 CUPS LOW-SODIUM VEGETABLE STOCK**

**3 SPRIGS THYME**

**1 CUP WHITE RICE**

**2 TBSP LOW-FAT GREEK YOGURT**

---

1. Heat the oil in a large pan or wok over a medium-high heat.
2. Add the scallions for a few minutes.
3. Now add the mushrooms and stir.
4. Add the stock, thyme and rice and cook until the liquid has been absorbed (25-30 minutes).
5. You will need to stir throughout to prevent the rice from sticking.
6. Top with the Greek yogurt to serve.

Per serving: Calories: 107; Fat: 4g (Saturated Fat: 1g); Carbohydrates: 15g; Fiber: 1g; Sugar: 2g; Sodium: 380mg; Protein: 4g

# MACARONI & CHEESE

**SERVES 4  /  PREP TIME: 5 MINUTES  /  COOK TIME: 30 MINUTES**

Creamy, bubbly and cheesy.

---

**1 1/2 CUPS MACARONI PASTA OR GLU-TEN-FREE EQUIVALENT**

**FOR THE CHEESE SAUCE:**

**1 TBSP UNSALTED BUTTER**

**1/8 CUP ALMOND MEAL**

**1 CUP SKIM MILK OR EQUIVALENT**

**1/2 CUP LOW-FAT COTTAGE CHEESE**

**1 TBSP FRESH PARSLEY, CHOPPED**

---

1. Cook the macaroni according to package guidelines.
2. Meanwhile, heat the butter in a small pan over a low-medium heat.
3. Tilt the pan towards you so that the butter melts only on the near side of the pan as much as possible.
4. Add the almond meal to the far side of the pan and slowly mix this into the melted butter using a wooden spoon.
5. Once a paste is formed, add the milk slowly and stir continuously for approximately 10-15 minutes or until the lumps disappear (don't worry, they will!)
6. Add the cottage cheese and stir thoroughly until lumps have dissolved again.
7. Drain the macaroni and mix into the cheese sauce.
8. Pour into an oven dish.
9. Broil under a medium heat for 10-15 minutes or until golden and bubbly.
10. Serve with a sprinkle of fresh parsley.

Per serving: Calories: 183.25; Fat: 7g (Saturated Fat: 2.25g); Carbohydrates: 20.5g; Fiber: 1.5g; Sugar: 4.5g; Sodium: 148.5mg; Protein: 9.25g

# ZUCCHINI MINT & CHIVE SOUP

**SERVES 2 / PREP TIME: 5 MINUTES / COOK TIME: 20 MINUTES**

Light and refreshing!

---

**1/2 CUP LOW-SODIUM VEGETABLE STOCK**

**1 CUP WATER**

**1 CUP ZUCCHINI, PEELED AND DICED**

**1 TBSP MINT, FRESHLY CHOPPED**

**1 TBSP FRESH CHIVES, CHOPPED**

---

1. Cut the carrot and zucchini into thin strips or batons.
2. Cook the noodles according to package directions.
3. Heat the oil in a skillet over a medium-high heat.
4. Add the carrots, zucchini, honey and five-spice.
5. Stir fry for 10 minutes.
6. Drain the noodles and add to the pan with the rest of the ingredients.
7. Serve hot and enjoy.

Per serving: Calories: 129; Fat: 4g (Saturated Fat: 0g); Carbohydrates: 21g; Fiber: 2g; Sugar: 6g; Sodium: 29mg; Protein: 4g; Potassium; 274mg

# VEGETABLE CHINESE-SPICED STIR FRY

**SERVES 4 / PREP TIME: 5 MINUTES / COOK TIME: 15 MINUTES**

A great vegetarian recipe for any meal.

---

1 MEDIUM CARROT, PEELED

1 SMALL ZUCCHINI, PEELED

1 CUP EGG NOODLES

1 TSP CANOLA OIL

1 TSP RAW HONEY

1 TSP CHINESE FIVE-SPICE

---

1. Cut the carrot and zucchini into thin strips or batons.
2. Cook the noodles according to package directions.
3. Heat the oil in a skillet over a medium-high heat.
4. Add the carrots, zucchini, honey and five-spice.
5. Stir fry for 10 minutes.
6. Drain the noodles and add to the pan with the rest of the ingredients.
7. Serve hot and enjoy.

Per serving: Calories: 129; Fat: 4g (Saturated Fat: 0g); Carbohydrates: 21g; Fiber: 2g; Sugar: 6g; Sodium: 29mg; Protein: 4g; Potassium; 274mg

# BUTTER NUT SQUASH RISOTTO

**SERVES 6 / PREP TIME: 10 MINUTES / COOK TIME: 30 MINUTES**

Packed with flavor and goodness.

---

**1 TBSP OLIVE OIL**

**1 CUP BUTTER NUT SQUASH, SKINLESS, DICED & STEAMED**

**2 CUPS UNCOOKED WHITE RICE**

**2 CUPS LOW SODIUM VEG STOCK**

**2 CUPS WATER**

**3 SPRIGS ROSEMARY**

---

1. Heat the oil in a skillet over a medium-high heat.
2. Add the steamed squash and heat through.
3. Now add the rice, stock, water and rosemary.
4. Cover and simmer for 20 minutes or until the stock is absorbed.
5. Stir throughout cooking.
6. Stir again and serve.

Per serving: Calories: 104; Fat: 2g (Saturated Fat: 0g); Carbohydrates: 18g; Fiber: 1g; Sugar: 1g; Sodium: 249mg; Protein: 2g

# RICE FIESTA

**SERVES 4 / PREP TIME: 5 MINUTES / COOK TIME: 20 MINUTES**

Simple yet scrumptious rice dish.

---

| | |
|---|---|
| **1 CUP WHITE RICE** | **1/2 CUP SILKEN TOFU, CUBED** |
| **1 TBSP COCONUT OIL** | **1 TSP BASIL, FRESHLY CHOPPED** |
| **1/2 CUP MUSHROOMS, SLICED** | **1 TSP CILANTRO, FRESHLY CHOPPED** |
| **1/2 CARROT, PEELED AND FINELY DICED** | |

---

1. Cook the rice according to package directions.
2. Meanwhile, heat the oil in a skillet over a medium-high heat.
3. Add the rest of the ingredients (minus the herbs) and sauté for 10-15 minutes.
4. Mix the vegetables through the rice and serve with the fresh herbs.

Per serving: Calories: 106; Fat: 5g (Saturated Fat: 3g); Carbohydrates: 13g; Fiber: 1g; Sugar: 1g; Sodium: 11mg; Protein: 3g

# SAG ALOO

**SERVES 4  /  PREP TIME: 5 MINUTES  /  COOK TIME: 35 MINUTES**

A little twist on the Indian favorite.

---

**2 MEDIUM WHITE POTATOES, PEELED AND CUBED**

**1 TSP ALLSPICE**

**1 TSP NUTMEG**

**1 TSP CINNAMON**

**1/2 CUP FROZEN SPINACH, THAWED**

---

1. Bring a pot of water to the boil and add the potato cubes.
2. Boil for 20-25 minutes or until soft (but not mushy).
3. Drain the potatoes.
4. Heat a skillet over a medium-high heat.
5. Add the potatoes and spices and sauté for 3-4 minutes.
6. Now add the spinach for 5-6 minutes or until hot through.
7. Serve hot.

Per serving: Calories: 50; Fat: 1g (Saturated Fat: 0g); Carbohydrates: 11g; Fiber: 2g; Sugar: 1g; Sodium: 27mg; Protein: 2g

# MUSHROOM NOODLES

**SERVES 2 / PREP TIME: 5 MINUTES / COOK TIME: 20 MINUTES**

A vegetarian take on a traditional dish.

---

1/4 CUP MUSHROOMS

1/4 CUP SPINACH

1 EGG

1/2 CUP LOW SODIUM VEGETABLE STOCK

1 CUP WATER

1 CUP EGG NOODLES

1 TSP CHINESE FIVE- SPICE

1 TBSP PARSLEY, FRESHLY CHOPPED

---

1. Cook mushrooms and spinach in a skillet for 10 minutes or until well cooked. Add a little oil if necessary to prevent sticking.
2. Meanwhile, boil the egg in a pot of boiling water for 5-6 minutes.
3. Rinse under the cold tap and remove the shell carefully.
4. Place veg and egg to one side.
5. In a pot, bring the stock and water to a simmer over a medium heat.
6. Add the noodles, spinach and mushrooms and lower the heat slightly.
7. Sprinkle in the Chinese five-spice.
8. Allow to simmer for 5-10 minutes or until noodles are thoroughly cooked.
9. Once piping hot, remove and serve with half a boiled egg each and a sprinkle of parsley.

Per serving: Calories: 162; Fat: 4g (Saturated Fat: 0.5g); Carbohydrates: 23g; Fiber: 2g; Sugar: 1g; Sodium: 122mg; Protein: 5.5g

# TOFU SCRAMBLE

**SERVES 2 / PREP TIME: 5 MINUTES / COOK TIME: 20 MINUTES**

Delicious vegetarian meal.

---

**1 TSP COCONUT OIL**

**1 CUP SILKEN TOFU, CUBED**

**1 TSP GINGER PASTE**

**1/4 CUP MUSHROOMS**

**1/4 CUP SPINACH**

---

1. Heat the coconut oil in a wok or non-stick skillet over a high heat.
2. Add the tofu and ginger paste and brown for 5-10 minutes.
3. Add the mushrooms and spinach for 10 minutes or until thoroughly cooked through.
4. Serve hot with your choice of rice or noodles.

Per serving: Calories: 101; Fat: 7g (Saturated Fat: 3g); Carbohydrates: 3g; Fiber: 1g; Sugar: 1g; Sodium: 14mg; Protein: 9g; Potassium; 209mg

# SOUPS AND STEWS

# TASTY TURKEY SOUP

**SERVES 8 / PREP TIME: 5 MINUTES / COOK TIME: 40 MINUTES**

Wholesome!

---

| | |
|---|---|
| 1 TSP OLIVE OIL | 1 BAY LEAF |
| 14OZ LEAN GROUND TURKEY MINCE | 1/4 CUP SCALLIONS, CHOPPED |
| 4 CUPS LOW SODIUM CHICKEN STOCK | 2 TSP HERBS DE PROVENCE |
| 1 MEDIUM CARROT, PEELED AND DICED | 1/2 CUP FROZEN SPINACH |

---

1. Heat the oil in a large pot over a medium-high heat.
2. Add the turkey mince and brown for 5 minutes.
3. Now add the rest of the ingredients, cover and simmer for 30-40 minutes.
4. Serve hot!

Per serving: Calories: 136; Fat: 7g (Saturated Fat: 2g); Carbohydrates: 4g; Fiber: 1g; Sugar: 1g; Sodium: 99mg; Protein: 16g

# ZUCCHINI & CHIVE SOUP

**SERVES 4 / PREP TIME: 5 MINUTES / COOK TIME: 10 MINUTES**

Light and refreshing!

---

**1/2 CUP LOW-SODIUM VEGETABLE STOCK**

**1 1/2 CUPS WATER**

**1 CUP ZUCCHINI, PEELED AND DICED**

**1 TBSP MINT, FRESHLY CHOPPED**

**1 TBSP FRESH CHIVES, CHOPPED**

---

1. Add the stock to a large pot over a medium heat and bring to a simmer.
2. Add the zucchini for 5-10 minutes or until thoroughly cooked through.
3. Now add the spinach and mint and cook for a further 5-10 minutes or until spinach is thoroughly cooked through.
4. Allow to cool slightly and blend in food processor until smooth.
5. Sprinkle in the chives and enjoy hot!

Per serving: Calories: 124; Fat: 5g (Saturated Fat: 1.5g); Carbohydrates: 6g; Fiber: 1.5g; Sugar: 3g; Sodium: 254mg; Protein: 2g

# LEAN CHICKEN & NOODLE SOUP

**SERVES 8 / PREP TIME: 5 MINUTES / COOK TIME: 40 MINUTES**

Great for colds!

---

12 OZ CHICKEN BREASTS, SKINLESS AND COOKED

2 TSP UNSALTED BUTTER

1 MEDIUM CARROT, PEELED AND CHOPPED

1/2 CUP SCALLIONS, CHOPPED

1 TSP DRIED SAGE

4 CUPS LOW SODIUM CHICKEN STOCK

1 CUP EGG NOODLES

---

1. Slice the cooked chicken. Note, use leftovers or precook the chicken under the broiler on a medium heat for 12-15 minutes.
2. Melt the butter in a large pot over a medium-high heat.
3. Sauté the carrot and scallions for 5 minutes.
4. Add seasoning, stock, noodles and chicken and simmer for 30-40 minutes.

Per serving: Calories: 100; Fat: 3g (Saturated Fat: 1g); Carbohydrates: 6; Fiber: 1g; Sugar: 1g; Sodium: 198mg; Protein: 13g

# HERBY CHICKEN STEW

**SERVES 8  /  PREP TIME: 5 MINUTES  /  COOK TIME: 4 HOURS**

Easy to prepare in the slow cooker - this stew is delicious.

---

**2 X 8OZ SKINLESS, BONELESS CHICKEN THIGHS, SLICED**

**1 MEDIUM SWEET POTATO, PEELED AND CHOPPED**

**1 TSP DRIED THYME**

**1 TSP DRIED SAGE**

**1 TSP DRIED PARSLEY**

**2 CUPS HOMEMADE TOMATO SAUCE**

**2 CUPS WATER**

**1 MEDIUM CARROT, PEELED AND CHOPPED**

**1 MEDIUM PARSNIP, PEELED AND CHOPPED**

---

1. Combine all of the ingredients in a slow cooker.
2. Cover and cook on a low heat for 8 hours or on a high heat setting for 4 hours.
3. Serve with your choice of rice.

Per serving: Calories: 147; Fat: 3g (Saturated Fat: 1g); Carbohydrates: 11g; Fiber: 2g; Sugar: 5g; Sodium: 305mg; Protein: 18g

# SLOW COOKED TURKEY STEW

**SERVES 8 / PREP TIME: 5 MINUTES / COOK TIME: 4 HOURS**

Another simple yet tasty dish.

---

**2 X 5OZ TURKEY BREASTS, SKINLESS**

**2 CUPS WATER**

**2 CUPS LOW SODIUM CHICKEN STOCK**

**1 BAY LEAF**

**1 TBSP LOW-SODIUM TOMATO PASTE**

**1 LARGE CARROT, CHOPPED**

**1 TBSP BALSAMIC VINEGAR**

---

1. Add all of the ingredients to a stock pot.
2. Cook on a low setting for 8 hours or overnight. Alternatively cook on high for 4 hours.
3. Shred the turkey (if it hasn't already flaked apart).
4. Portion up and enjoy.

Per serving: Calories: 45; Fat: 1g (Saturated Fat: 0g); Carbohydrates: 2g; Fiber: 0g; Sugar: 1g; Sodium:36mg; Protein: 8g

# VEGETARIAN CASSEROLE

**SERVES 6 / PREP TIME: 5 MINUTES / COOK TIME: 4 HOURS**

Hearty and warming.

---

2 MEDIUM CARROTS, PEELED AND CHOPPED

2 MEDIUM TURNIPS, PEELED AND CHOPPED

2 MEDIUM PARSNIPS, PEELED AND CHOPPED

2 CUPS LOW-SODIUM VEG STOCK

2 CUPS WATER

1 TBSP DRIED THYME

1 TBSP DRIED TARRAGON

1 TBSP GINGER, GROUND

1 TSP NUTMEG, GROUND

1 TSP CINNAMON

---

1. Add all of the ingredients to the slow cooker.
2. Cook on a low setting for 8 hours or overnight. Alternatively cook on high for 4 hours.
3. Enjoy.

Per serving: Calories: 37; Fat: 1g (Saturated Fat: 0g); Carbohydrates: 7g; Fiber: 2g; Sugar: 2g; Sodium: 259mg; Protein: 1g

# SLOW COOKED PUMPKIN & SPINACH STEW

**SERVES 6 / PREP TIME: 5 MINUTES / COOK TIME: 4 HOURS**

Hearty and warming.

---

**2 CUPS FRESH PUMPKIN**

**2 CUPS SPINACH**

**1 CUP LOW SODIUM TOMATO SAUCE**

**3 CUPS WATER**

**2 SPRIGS ROSEMARY**

**1 TSP DRIED THYME**

**1 TSP CINNAMON**

---

1. Add all of the ingredients to the slow cooker (except spinach).
2. Cook on a low setting for 8 hours or overnight. Alternatively cook on high for 4 hours.
3. 20 minutes before serving, add the spinach.
4. Enjoy.

Per serving: Calories: 37; Fat: 1g (Saturated Fat: 0g); Carbohydrates: 7g; Fiber: 2g; Sugar: 3g; Sodium: 34; Protein: 2g

# PEANUT CHICKEN STEW

**SERVES 8 / PREP TIME: 5 MINUTES / COOK TIME: 4 HOURS**

Trust this one - it's good!

---

**2 TBSP PEANUT BUTTER**

**4 X 4OZ CHICKEN THIGHS, SKINLESS & BONELESS**

**2 CUPS LOW-SODIUM TOMATO SAUCE**

**2 CUPS WATER**

**1 TBSP ALLSPICE**

**1 TSP GROUND NUTMEG**

---

1. Add all of the ingredients to the slow cooker.
2. Cook on a low setting for 8 hours or overnight. Alternatively cook on high for 4 hours.
3. Enjoy.

Per serving: Calories: 140; Fat: 7g (Saturated Fat: 2g); Carbohydrates: 4g; Fiber: 1g; Sugar: 2g; Sodium: 275mg; Protein: 15g

# ROSEMARY CHICKEN & RICE CASSEROLE

**SERVES 8 / PREP TIME: 10 MINUTES / COOK TIME: 4 HOURS**

Hearty and warming.

---

**1 TBSP OLIVE OIL**

**1 TBSP ROSEMARY, DRIED & CRUSHED**

**4 X 4OZ CHICKEN THIGHS, SKINLESS & BONELESS**

**2 CUPS WATER**

**2 CUPS LOW-SODIUM CHICKEN STOCK**

**2 CUPS SPINACH, WASHED**

**2 CUPS UNCOOKED WHITE RICE**

---

1. Mix the olive oil and herbs together and marinate the chicken in a sealed container in the refrigerator for as long as possible (up to overnight).
2. When ready to cook, add all of the ingredients to the slow cooker, except the spinach and rice.
3. Cook on a low setting for 8 hours or overnight. Alternatively cook on high for 4 hours.
4. 20 minutes before serving, add the rice.
5. 10 minutes before serving, add the spinach to wilt.
6. Stir through and serve hot.

Per serving: Calories: 184; Fat: 7g (Saturated Fat: 2g); Carbohydrates: 14g; Fiber: 1g; Sugar: 0g; Sodium: 302mg; Protein: 17g

# SHRIMP CASSEROLE

**SERVES 8 / PREP TIME: 5 MINUTES / COOK TIME: 1 HOUR**

Hearty and warming.

---

2 CUPS LOW-SODIUM VEG STOCK

1/2 CUP LOW-SODIUM TOMATO SAUCE

1/2 CUP ACORN SQUASH, PEELED AND DICED

1 MEDIUM CARROT, PEELED AND DICED

1 TSP THYME

1 BAY LEAF

16 OZ SHRIMP, FULLY DEFROSTED & DE-VEINED

---

1. Add all of the ingredients into the slow cooker.
2. Cook on a low setting for 1 hour.
3. Alternatively cook on high for 30 minutes.
4. Enjoy.

Per serving: Calories: 87; Fat: 1g (Saturated Fat: 0g); Carbohydrates: 3g; Fiber: 0g; Sugar: 1g; Sodium: 379mg; Protein: 15g

# POTATO & CHIVE SOUP

**SERVES 4 / PREP TIME: 5 MINUTES / COOK TIME: 40 MINUTES**

A deliciously thick vegetable soup.

---

1 TBSP UNSALTED BUTTER/OLIVE OIL

4 SMALL WHITE POTATOES, PEELED AND CUBED

5 TBSP CHIVES, FRESHLY CHOPPED

1/4 CUP SCALLIONS, FINELY CHOPPED

1 CUP LOW-SODIUM VEG STOCK

1 CUP WATER

1 BAY LEAF

4 TBSP LOW-FAT GREEK YOGURT

---

1. Melt the butter/oil in a large pot over a medium-high heat.
2. Sauté the potatoes, chives and scallions for 5 minutes.
3. Add the rest of the ingredients (except yogurt) and simmer for 30-40 minutes.
4. Allow to cool slightly then blitz in a food processor until smooth.
5. Serve hot with 1 tbsp Greek yogurt stirred through.

Per serving: Calories: 127; Fat: 3g (Saturated Fat: 2g); Carbohydrates: 22g; Fiber: 2g; Sugar: 2g; Sodium: 424mg; Protein: 4g

# INDONESIAN BROTH

**SERVES 8 / PREP TIME: 5 MINUTES / COOK TIME: 25 MINUTES**

Served with a boiled egg - this is a real winner!

---

1 TBSP COCONUT OIL

1 LARGE CARROT, PEELED AND DICED

1 TBSP ALLSPICE

1 TSP CINNAMON

2 CUPS LOW-SODIUM CHICKEN STOCK

4 CUPS WATER

1 CUP EGG NOODLES

16OZ COOKED AND SHREDDED CHICKEN

BREAST

1 CUP MUSHROOMS, WELL-COOKED

4 HARD BOILED EGGS

2 TBSP CILANTRO, FRESHLY CHOPPED

---

1. Heat the oil in a large pot over a medium-high heat.
2. Sauté the carrots for 3-4 minutes.
3. Add the seasoning, stock, water, noodles and chicken.
4. Cover and simmer for 15 minutes.
5. Now add the mushrooms and continue to simmer for a further 10 minutes.
6. Once piping hot, remove and serve with the halved boiled eggs, a sprinkle of cilantro and a squeeze of lemon juice.

Per serving: Calories: 176; Fat: 7g (Saturated Fat: 3g); Carbohydrates: 6g; Fiber: 1g; Sugar: 1g; Sodium: 332mg; Protein: 22g

# SPRING GREENS SOUP

**SERVES 4 / PREP TIME: 5 MINUTES / COOK TIME: 10 MINUTES**

Light and refreshing!

---

1 TBSP OLIVE OIL

1/2 CUP CHOPPED SCALLIONS

1 CUP GREEN ZUCCHINI, PEELED, CENTRE REMOVED & DICED

2 CUPS LOW-SODIUM VEGETABLE STOCK

2 CUPS WATER

1 CUP SPINACH, WASHED

2 TBSP MINT, FRESHLY CHOPPED

---

1. Heat the oil in a large pot over a medium-high heat.
2. Add the scallions and zucchini for 1-2 minutes.
3. Add the stock and water; bring to a simmer.
4. Now add the spinach and cook for 5-10 minutes or until vegetables are thoroughly cooked through.
5. Allow to cool slightly and blend in a food processor until smooth.
6. Serve with a little butter stirred into the soup (optional) and a sprinkling of fresh mint leaves.

Per serving: Calories: 92; Fat: 7g (Saturated Fat: 2g); Carbohydrates: 7g; Fiber: 2g; Sugar: 2g; Sodium: 409mg; Protein: 3g

# BRILLIANT BEET & SWEET POTATO SOUP

**SERVES 4 / PREP TIME: 5 MINUTES / COOK TIME: 30 MINUTES**

A great and simple soup dish.

---

**1 TBSP OLIVE OIL**

**1 LARGE SWEET POTATO, PEELED AND CUBED**

**2 BEETS, COOKED AND CUBED**

**1 TSP DRIED DILL**

**2 CUPS LOW-SODIUM VEG STOCK**

**1 CUP WATER**

**4 TBSP LOW-FAT GREEK YOGURT**

---

1. Heat the oil in a large pot over a medium-high heat.
2. Add the sweet potatoes and beets for 2 minutes.
3. Now add the dill, stock and water and bring to a simmer for 25-30 minutes.
4. Swirl through 1 tbsp Greek yogurt in each bowl to serve..

Per serving: Calories: 93; Fat: 4g (Saturated Fat: 1g); Carbohydrates: 12g; Fiber: 2g; Sugar: 5g; Sodium: 406mg; Protein: 4g

# CARROT & GINGER SOUP

**SERVES 5 / PREP TIME: 10 MINUTES / COOK TIME: 35 MINUTES**

Zingy and aromatic!

---

2 CUPS LOW-SODIUM VEG STOCK

2 CUPS WATER

1 MEDIUM PARSNIP, PEELED AND CHOPPED

4 MEDIUM CARROTS, PEELED AND CHOPPED

1 TBSP GROUND GINGER

1 TSP GROUND NUTMEG

---

1. Over a medium-high heat, bring the stock and water to a simmer in a large pot.
2. Add the carrots and parsnips along with the ginger.
3. Simmer for 30-35 minutes or until vegetables are very soft.
4. Allow to cool slightly, then blend in a food processor until smooth.
5. Serve with a sprinkle of nutmeg.

Per serving: Calories: 42; Fat: 0g (Saturated Fat: 0g); Carbohydrates: 9g; Fiber: 2g; Sugar: 3g; Sodium: 326mg; Protein: 2g

# TOMATO SOUP

**SERVES 4 / PREP TIME: 10 MINUTES / COOK TIME: 20 MINUTES**

A wonderfully light tomato soup.

---

2 SLICES THICK-CUT WHITE BREAD (SLIGHTLY STALE)

2 CUPS CANNED TOMATOES, SKINLESS

1 TSP STEVIA POWDER

1 TBSP BALSAMIC VINEGAR

2 TBSP BASIL, FRESHLY TORN

4 TSP OLIVE OIL

---

1. Tear the bread into croûton pieces and soak in warm water.
2. Press the tomatoes through a strainer or sieve to get rid of any seeds or pulp.
3. Heat a pot on a low heat and add the tomatoes, stevia and balsamic vinegar.
4. Add a little water to bulk out if needed.
5. Allow to simmer for 10-15 minutes.
6. Sprinkle with basil and stir in 1 tsp olive oil in each bowl to serve.

Per serving: Calories: 67; Fat: 2g (Saturated Fat: 0g); Carbohydrates: 13g; Fiber: 1g; Sugar: 5g; Sodium: 320mg; Protein: 2g

# CREAMY MUSHROOM SOUP

**SERVES 4 / PREP TIME: 5 MINUTES / COOK TIME: 30 MINUTES**

A comforting bowl on a Winter's night!

| | |
|---|---|
| 1 TBSP UNSALTED BUTTER | 2 CUPS LOW-SODIUM VEG STOCK |
| 1 SPRIG THYME | 1 CUP WATER |
| 2 CUPS MUSHROOMS, CHOPPED | 2 TBSP LOW-FAT GREEK YOGURT |
| 1 TBSP ALL-PURPOSE WHITE FLOUR (GF IF NEEDED) | 1 TSP GROUND NUTMEG |
| | 1 TSP TARRAGON, FRESHLY CHOPPED |

1. Melt the butter in a large pot over a medium-low heat.
2. Add the thyme and stir for 5 minutes.
3. Turn the heat up slightly and add the mushrooms for 3 minutes.
4. Sprinkle the flour over the mushrooms and stir for 2 minutes.
5. Add the stock and water to the pot.
6. Bring to the boil, turn down the heat and allow to simmer for 20 minutes.
7. Remove the thyme and allow to cool slightly.
8. Blitz in a food processor until smooth.
9. Return to the pot and add the Greek yogurt, nutmeg and tarragon before stirring for 2-3 minutes.
10. Enjoy!

Per serving: Calories: 54; Fat: 3g (Saturated Fat: 2g); Carbohydrates: 4g; Fiber: 1g; Sugar: 2g; Sodium: 376mg; Protein: 3g

# MUSHROOM BROTH

**SERVES 5 / PREP TIME: 5 MINUTES / COOK TIME: 35 MINUTES**

A lovely broth that can be enjoyed as a soup or as a stock for cooking.

---

1 TBSP UNSALTED BUTTER

1/2 CUP SCALLIONS, CHOPPED

2 MEDIUM CARROTS, PEELED AND CHOPPED

3 CUPS MUSHROOMS, CHOPPED

1 TSP DRIED THYME

2 CUPS LOW-SODIUM VEG STOCK

1 CUP WATER

---

1. Melt the butter in a pot over a medium-low heat.
2. Add the carrots and scallions and stir.
3. Sauté for 10 minutes.
4. Add the mushrooms to the pot and stir.
5. Add the thyme, stock and water and then simmer for 20 minutes.
6. Allow to cool slightly before blending in a food processor until smooth.
7. Enjoy!

Per serving: Calories: 44; Fat: 3g (Saturated Fat: 1g); Carbohydrates: 4g; Fiber: 1g; Sugar: 2g; Sodium: 309mg; Protein: 2g

# ROOT VEG & GINGER SOUP

**SERVES 5 / PREP TIME: 5 MINUTES / COOK TIME: 30 MINUTES**

Ginger is great for upset stomachs and really spices up the veg in this soup!

---

1 TBSP OLIVE OIL

1/2 CUP SCALLIONS, CHOPPED

1 TSP GROUND GINGER

1 TSP CUMIN

1 TSP GROUND NUTMEG

2 MEDIUM PARSNIPS, PEELED AND DICED

2 MEDIUM TURNIPS, PEELED AND DICED

2 CUPS LOW-SODIUM VEG STOCK

1 CUP WATER

4 TBSP LOW-FAT GREEK YOGURT (OPTIONAL)

---

1. Heat the oil in a large pot over a medium-low heat.
2. Add the scallions, ginger, cumin and nutmeg and stir for 2 minutes.
3. Add the parsnips and turnips and stir well to mix in the spices.
4. Add the stock and water to the pot and simmer for 20 minutes or until vegetables are soft.
5. Remove from heat and allow to cool.
6. Blitz in a food processor until smooth.
7. Return to the pot to warm through.
8. Serve with a swirl of Greek yogurt.
9. Enjoy!

Per serving: Calories: 69; Fat: 3g (Saturated Fat: 0g); Carbohydrates: 9g; Fiber: 2g; Sugar: 3g; Sodium: 263mg; Protein: 3g

# HONEY BUTTER NUT SQUASH SOUP

**SERVES 5 / PREP TIME: 10 MINUTES / COOK TIME: 55 MINUTES**

Sweet and savory Autumnal bliss!

---

**1 CUP BUTTER NUT SQUASH, PEELED, DE-SEEDED AND CUBED**

**2 TBSP HONEY**

**1 TBSP PARSLEY, DRIED**

**2 CUPS LOW-SODIUM VEG STOCK**

---

1. Preheat the oven to 350°f/170°c/Gas Mark 4.
2. Layer the squash onto a non-stick baking tray.
3. Drizzle over the honey and sprinkle over the parsley.
4. Toss to coat.
5. Bake in the oven for 35-40 minutes and remove.
6. Bring the stock to a simmer on a medium-low heat.
7. Add the cubed squash to the stock and simmer for 15 minutes.
8. Remove from heat and allow to cool.
9. Blitz in a food processor until smooth.
10. Return to a low heat to warm through and serve.

Per serving: Calories: 57; Fat: 0g (Saturated Fat: 0g); Carbohydrates: 14g; Fiber: 1g; Sugar: 10g; Sodium: 376mg; Protein: 2g

# THAI SEAFOOD BROTH

**SERVES 4  /  PREP TIME: 15 MINUTES /  COOK TIME: 25 MINUTES**

Fresh and zingy!

---

1 TBSP COCONUT OIL

10OZ SHRIMP, DE-VEINED

1 TBSP OF LEMONGRASS, FINELY DICED

1 CUP  LOW-SODIUM CHICKEN STOCK

1 CUP WATER

1/4 CUP SCALLIONS, CHOPPED

1 TBSP BASIL, FRESHLY CHOPPED

---

1. Heat the oil in a large pot over a medium heat.
2. Add the shrimp and lemongrass and cook for 6-7 minutes or until pink.
3. Add the chicken stock and water; bring to a simmer.
4. Add the rest of the ingredients and simmer for 15 minutes.
5. Serve!

Per serving: Calories: 95; Fat: 5g (Saturated Fat: 3g); Carbohydrates: 3g; Fiber: 0g; Sugar: 0g; Sodium: 486mg; Protein: 11g

# SIDES & SNACKS

# SPICED SWEET POTATO THINS

**SERVES 6 / PREP TIME: 5 MINUTES / COOK TIME: 15 MINUTES**

Delicious side or snack!

---

**2 SWEET POTATOES, PEELED AND FINELY SLICED**

**1 TBSP CILANTRO, FRESHLY CHOPPED**

**1 TSP GROUND CUMIN**

**1/2 TSP GROUND NUTMEG**

**1 TSP GROUND GINGER**

**1 TBSP OLIVE OIL**

---

1. Preheat the broiler to a medium-high heat.
2. Layer the potato slices on a lined baking tray.
3. Mix the herbs and spices with the oil in a separate bowl.
4. Cover the potato slices and toss to coat.
5. Broil for 10-15 minutes or until cooked through.

Per serving: Calories: 58; Fat: 3g (Saturated Fat: 0g); Carbohydrates: 8g; Fiber: 1g; Sugar: 3g; Sodium: 15mg; Protein: 1g

# PARSLEY TURNIP MASH

**SERVES 5  /  PREP TIME: 5 MINUTES  /  COOK TIME: 20 MINUTES**

Delicious side to your favorite meat or fish.

---

**4 TURNIPS, PEELED AND DICED**

**1 TBSP PARSLEY, FRESHLY CHOPPED**

**1 TBSP UNSALTED BUTTER**

---

1. Add the turnips to a pot of water (4 cups) on a high heat.
2. Bring to the boil and then turn down the heat slightly.
3. Allow to simmer for 20 minutes or until turnips are soft.
4. Drain the turnips and mash with a potato masher or fork.
5. Add the butter and parsley and mash together.
6. Serve hot!

Per serving: Calories: 41; Fat: 1g (Saturated Fat: 1g); Carbohydrates: 5g; Fiber: 2g; Sugar: 3g; Sodium: 16mg; Protein: 1

# SWEET POTATO MASH

**SERVES 4 / PREP TIME: 5 MINUTES / COOK TIME: 20 MINUTES**

Scrumptious!

---

**2 SWEET POTATOES, PEELED AND CHOPPED**

**1 TBSP OLIVE OIL**

**1 TBSP LOW-FAT GREEK YOGURT**

**1 TBSP CILANTRO, FRESHLY CHOPPED**

---

1. Place the sweet potatoes and olive oil in a microwavable zip lock bag.
2. Place this into the microwave for 20 minutes. Alternatively, boil in a pot for 25 minutes.
3. Remove the sweet potato from the microwave and very carefully unzip the bag (it will be steaming hot).
4. Pop the sweet potato into a large bowl and mash with a fork or potato masher.
5. Stir through the yogurt and season with fresh herbs.

Per serving: Calories: 83; Fat: 3g (Saturated Fat: 0g); Carbohydrates: 12g; Fiber: 2g; Sugar: 4g; Sodium: 22mg; Protein: 2g

# ACORN SQUASH SIDE

**SERVES 6 / PREP TIME: 5 MINUTES / COOK TIME: 20 MINUTES**

A delicious dish.

---

1 ACORN SQUASH, PEELED AND CUBED

1 TBSP OLIVE OIL

1 TBSP PARSLEY, FRESHLY CHOPPED

4 SCALLIONS, CHOPPED

---

1. Add the squash cubes to a pot of water on a high heat.
2. Bring to the boil and then turn down the heat slightly.
3. Allow to simmer for 20 minutes or until squash is soft.
4. Drain the squash and add to a serving bowl with the rest of the ingredients and mix.
5. Serve hot!

Per serving: Calories: 52; Fat: 2g (Saturated Fat: 0g); Carbohydrates: 8g; Fiber: 1g; Sugar: 0g; Sodium: 4mg; Protein: 1g

# BAKED SQUASH LOAF

**SERVES 15 SLICES / PREP TIME: 20 MINUTES / COOK TIME: 50 MINUTES**

Delicious to mop up a stew or with your favorite spread!

---

1 BUTTER NUT SQUASH , PEELED AND CUBED

1/4 CUP COLD WATER

1 TSP PARSLEY

1 TSP THYME

2 TSP BAKING POWDER

2 TBSP OLIVE OIL

2 CUPS WHITE FLOUR (GF IF NEEDED)

---

1. Preheat the oven to 400°f/190°c/Gas Mark 5.
2. Add the squash cubes to a pot of water (enough to cover the squash) on a high heat.
3. Bring to the boil and then turn down the heat slightly.
4. Allow to simmer for 20 minutes or until squash is soft.
5. Drain the squash and add to a serving bowl and mash with a potato masher or fork.
6. Mix all of the ingredients together until a dough-like consistency is formed.
7. Knead the dough on a lightly floured surface until it is soft and spongy.
8. Shape the dough into a round loaf and place on a baking tray.
9. Score the top with a sharp knife in a pattern of your choice.
10. Bake for 35 minutes and then remove and allow to cool on a wired rack.
11. Slice with a bread knife and enjoy.

Per serving: Calories: 118; Fat: 2g (Saturated Fat: 0g); Carbohydrates: 24g; Fiber: 2g; Sugar: 2g; Sodium: 69mg; Protein: 3g

# HONEY ROASTED BEETS

**SERVES 4 / PREP TIME: 5 MINUTES / COOK TIME: 40 MINUTES**

A tempting snack.

---

**2 WHOLE BEETS, SCRUBBED AND SLICED**
**2 TBSP HONEY**

---

1. Preheat the oven to 375°f/190°c/Gas Mark 5.
2. Heat the honey on a medium heat in a skillet.
3. Add the beetroot to the skillet for a few minutes.
4. Transfer all ingredients to a baking tray, cover with foil and roast in the oven for 30-40 minutes.
5. When the beets are soft, remove and serve.

Per serving: Calories: 37; Fat: 0g (Saturated Fat: 0g); Carbohydrates: 10g; Fiber: 0g; Sugar: 10g; Sodium: 10mg; Protein: 0g

# YELLOW SQUASH DIP

**SERVES 6 / PREP TIME: 5-10 MINUTES / COOK TIME: 25 MINUTES**

Another tasty dip!

---

**2 CUPS YELLOW SQUASH, PEELED AND CUBED**

**1 TBSP OLIVE OIL**

**1 TSP PARSLEY**

**1 TSP THYME**

**1 TSP CUMIN**

---

1. Add the squash cubes to a pot of water (to cover squash) on a high heat.
2. Bring to the boil and then turn down the heat slightly.
3. Allow to simmer for 25 minutes or until squash is soft.
4. Drain the squash and add to a food processor with the rest of the ingredients.
5. Blitz until a smooth consistency is formed.

Per serving: Calories: 34; Fat: 3g (Saturated Fat: 0g); Carbohydrates: 3g; Fiber: 1g; Sugar: 2g; Sodium: 2mg; Protein: 1g

# BROTHS AND CONDIMENTS

# LOW-SODIUM CHICKEN STOCK

**SERVES 8 CUPS  /  PREP TIME: 5 MINUTES  /  COOK TIME: 3-4 HOURS**

Delicious stock that can be used in many of the recipes in this cookbook!

| | |
|---|---|
| **BONES OF 1 WHOLE CHICKEN** | **8 CUPS WATER** |
| **1/2 CUP SCALLIONS, CHOPPED** | **1 BAY LEAF** |
| **1/2 CUP CARROTS, PEELED AND CHOPPED** | **1 ZUCCHINI, PEELED AND CHOPPED** |
| **2 TBSP THYME** | |

1. Add all ingredients to a large pot on a medium heat and simmer for 3-4 hours.
2. Alternatively add to a slow cooker and cook on low for 12 hours.
3. Strain the stock through a fine sieve.
4. Allow to cool and then add to a sealed container in the refrigerator.
5. Use a spoon or knife to skim away any fat from the top before using or heat through thoroughly for a lovely broth to sip on.
6. You can freeze this in portions for up to 2-3 weeks and allow to defrost before use.

Hint: As homemade stock is high in calories and good fats but low in fiber, it can be sipped on throughout the day. Just don't forget to include in your daily calculations!

Please note: Each serving should be no more than 1/2 cup. If using in dishes, allocate 1/2 cup stock per person and use water to combine.

Per serving (1/2 cup) approx: Calories: 126; Fat: 7g (Saturated Fat: 2g); Carbohydrates: 1.25g; Fiber: 0g; Sugar: 0.5g; Sodium: 50.5mg; Protein: 13.5g

# VERY SIMPLE VEGETABLE STOCK

**SERVES 8 CUPS / PREP TIME: 5 MINUTES / COOK TIME: 3-4 HOURS**

A light stock for adding to vegetable or meat dishes.

---

| | |
|---|---|
| 1 CUP CARROTS, PEELED AND SLICED | 2 TSP ROSEMARY, CHOPPED |
| 1 CELERY STALK, CHOPPED | 1 BAY LEAF |
| 1 CUP MUSHROOMS, SLICED | 1 TSP CUMIN |
| 8 CUPS WATER | |
| 1 TSP SEA SALT | |
| 1 TSP PARSLEY | |

---

1. Add all ingredients to a large pot on a medium heat and simmer for 3-4 hours.
2. Alternatively add to a slow cooker and cook on low for 12 hours.
3. Strain the stock through a fine sieve.
4. Allow to cool and then add to a sealed container in the refrigerator.
5. Use a spoon or knife to skim away any fat from the top before using or heat through thoroughly for a lovely broth to sip on.
6. You can freeze this in portions for up to 2-3 weeks and allow to defrost before use.

Hint: As homemade stock is high in calories and good fats but low in fiber, it can be sipped on throughout the day. Just don't forget to include in your daily calculations!

Please note: Each serving should be no more than 1/2 cup. If using in dishes, allocate 1/2 cup stock per person and use water to combine.

Per serving (1/2 cup) approx: Calories: 9; Fat: 0g (Saturated Fat: 0g); Carbohydrates: 1.5g; Fiber: 0.5g; Sugar: 1g; Sodium: 50mg; Protein: 0g

# FISH BROTH

Lovely in Thai curries, fish stew or even a seafood paella!

---

**8 CUPS SHELLFISH (TRIMMINGS ARE FINE - ASK AT YOUR LOCAL FISHMONGER OR SUPERMARKET)**

**1/4 CUP SCALLIONS, CHOPPED**

**10 CUPS WATER**

**1 CELERY STALK, CHOPPED**

**1 TSP PARSLEY**

**1 TSP CILANTRO**

**3 CARROTS, PEELED AND CHOPPED**

---

1. Add all of the ingredients to a large pot over a medium heat.
2. Simmer for 3-4 hours. Alternatively use a slow cooker to free you from the kitchen and simmer on low overnight).
3. Strain the broth through a sieve.
4. Allow to cool and store in a sealable container in the fridge for 2-3 days or in the freezer for 2-3 weeks.

Approx. per cup: Calories: 69; Fat: 1g (Saturated Fat: 0g); Carbohydrates: 7g; Fiber: 1g; Sugar: 3g; Sodium: 90mg; Protein: 1g

# BONE BROTH

**SERVES 8 CUPS / PREP TIME: 5 MINUTES / COOK TIME: 3-4 HOURS**

You can add this to soups or stews for a rich taste, or simply sip from a mug throughout the day.

| | |
|---|---|
| **5 BEEF BONES** | **1 TSP CINNAMON** |
| **1 CUP CARROTS, CHOPPED** | **1 CELERY STALK, CHOPPED** |
| **1 TSP SEA SALT** | **10 CUPS WATER** |
| **1 BAY LEAF** | |
| **1 TSP NUTMEG** | |

1. Add all ingredients to a large pot on a medium heat and simmer for 3-4 hours.
2. Alternatively add to a slow cooker and cook on low for 12 hours.
3. Strain the broth through a fine sieve.
4. Allow to cool and then add to a sealed container in the refrigerator.
5. Use a spoon or knife to skim away any fat that has stored as a layer on the top.
6. You can freeze this in portions for up to 2-3 weeks and allow to defrost before use.

Please note: Each serving should be no more than 1/2 cup. If using in dishes, allocate 1/2 cup stock per person and use water to combine.

Per serving (1/2 cup) approx: Calories: 34.5; Fat: 2g (Saturated Fat: 1g); Carbohydrates: 0.5g; Fiber: 0g; Sugar: 0g; Sodium: 45mg; Protein: 3g

# TERRIFIC TOMATO SAUCE

**SERVES 20 / PREP TIME: 15 MINUTES / COOK TIME: 10 MINUTES**

Can be used with many of the recipes in this cookbook.

---

**5 CUPS LARGE VERY RIPE TOMATOES**

**1 TSP BASIL**

---

1. Cover the tomatoes with boiling water in a large bowl.
2. Leave for 3 minutes and drain.
3. Rinse with cold water before peeling skins off.
4. Quarter and de-seed tomatoes with a knife and then press the rest through a strainer or sieve to get rid of any pulp.
5. Do the same with the seeds from earlier to get as much juice as you can from them!
6. Add to a small pan on a medium heat and sprinkle with the herbs.
7. Allow to simmer for 10-15 minutes or until hot through.
8. Alternatively serve cold!

Per serving: Calories: 20; Fat: 0g (Saturated Fat: 0g); Carbohydrates: 4g; Fiber: 1g; Sugar: 2g; Sodium: 10mg; Protein: 1g

# WHITE SAUCE

**SERVES 5 / PREP TIME: 15 MINUTES / COOK TIME: 10 MINUTES**

A healthy white sauce to use with the recipes in this book or your own recipes!

---

**1 TBSP UNSALTED BUTTER**

**1OZ WHITE FLOUR (GF IF NEEDED)/AL-MOND MEAL**

**1 CUP SKIM MILK OR EQUIVALENT**

---

1. Heat the butter in a small pan over a low-medium heat.
2. Tilt the pan towards you so that the butter melts only on the near side of the pan as much as possible.
3. Add the flour to the far side of the pan and slowly mix this into the melted butter using a wooden spoon.
4. Once a paste is formed, add the milk slowly and stir continuously for approximately 10-15 minutes or until the lumps disappear (don't worry, they will!)

Per serving: Calories: 58; Fat: 2g (Saturated Fat: 1g); Carbohydrates: 7g; Fiber: 0g; Sugar: 3g; Sodium: 21mg; Protein: 2g

# GINGERED PURÉE

**SERVES 10 / PREP TIME: 5 MINUTES / COOK TIME: N/A**

Add to your stir-fries, poultry or even yogurts for a bit of a kick!

---

**2 WHOLE GINGER ROOT, PEELED AND SLICED**

**1 CUP WATER**

---

1. Add the ginger and water to a food processor until smooth.
2. Strain through a sieve.
3. Keep in a sealed container in the fridge for 2-3 days or add to an ice cube tray and simple pop into your dishes to add a ginger taste!

Per serving: Calories: 4; Fat: 0g (Saturated Fat: 0g); Carbohydrates: 0g; Fiber: 0g; Sugar: 0g; Sodium: 0mg; Protein: 0g

# GASTRO GRAVY

**SERVES 8  /  PREP TIME: 15 MINUTES / COOK TIME: 15 MINUTES**

You can feel confident serving this gravy with your roast chicken!

---

**1 TBSP OLIVE OIL**

**1/4 CUP SCALLIONS, FINELY CHOPPED**

**4 CUPS LOW-SODIUM CHICKEN STOCK**

**1 TSP PARSLEY**

---

1.  Add the oil to a pot over a medium heat.
2.  Add the scallions for 1-2 minutes.
3.  Add the rest of the ingredients and allow to simmer for 5-10 minutes or until it thickens.

Per serving: Calories: 146; Fat: 9g (Saturated Fat: 2g); Carbohydrates: 1g; Fiber: 0g; Sugar: 0g; Sodium: 51mg; Protein: 13g

# PEAR SAUCE

**SERVES 8 / PREP TIME: 5 MINUTES / COOK TIME: 10 MINUTES**

This is great swirled into your breakfast or served with cooked meats.

---

**2 CUPS PEARS, PEELED AND CHOPPED**

**1 TBSP SKIM MILK OR EQUIVALENT**

**1/2 TSP GROUND NUTMEG**

**1/2 TSP CINNAMON**

---

1. Steam the chopped pears over a steamer on a medium-high heat for 10 minutes.
2. Add with the rest of the ingredients to a food processor until smooth.
3. If you don't have a processor, cook for an extra 5 minutes and mash with a fork before passing through a sieve and adding the rest of the ingredients.
4. Serve right away or store in a sealable container in the fridge for 2-3 days.
5. Alternatively store in an ice cube tray and pop out to thaw before you need it.

Per serving: Calories: 39; Fat: 0g (Saturated Fat: 0g); Carbohydrates: 10g; Fiber: 1g; Sugar: 8g; Sodium: 3mg; Protein: 0g

# HARVEST PURÉE

**SERVES 10 / PREP TIME: 5 MINUTES / COOK TIME: 10 MINUTES**

Delicious with crackers or breads or over your cooked meats and veg.

---

**2 CUPS ACORN SQUASH, PEELED AND CUBED AND STEAMED**

**1/2 CUP COOKED COUSCOUS**

**1/4 CUP APPLESAUCE**

---

1. Add the ingredients to a food processor until smooth.
2. Serve right away or store in a sealable container in the fridge for 2-3 days.
3. Alternatively store in an ice cube tray and pop out to thaw before you need it.

Per serving: Calories: 45; Fat: 0g (Saturated Fat: 0g); Carbohydrates: 10g; Fiber: 1g; Sugar: 1g; Sodium: 2mg; Protein: 1g

# MANGO CHUTNEY

**SERVES 10 / PREP TIME: 5 MINUTES / COOK TIME: 20 MINUTES**

Tastes great!

---

**1 RIPE MANGO, PEELED AND CUBED**

**1/2 CUP WATER**

**1 TSP CILANTRO, FRESHLY CHOPPED**

---

1. Steam the mango cubes over a medium-high heat for 20 minutes.
2. Add to a food processor with the water until smooth.
3. Season with cilantro.
4. Serve right away or store in a sealable container in the fridge for 2-3 days.
5. Alternatively store in an ice cube tray and pop out to thaw before you need it.

Per serving: Calories: 14; Fat: 0g (Saturated Fat: 0g); Carbohydrates: 4g; Fiber: 0g; Sugar: 3g; Sodium: 4mg; Protein: 0g

# PEACH SAUCE

**SERVES 10 / PREP TIME: 5 MINUTES / COOK TIME: 15 MINUTES**

A lovely breakfast addition or served with poultry.

---

**5 RIPE PEACHES, PEELED**

**1/2 TSP GINGER, GRATED**

**1/2 TSP STEVIA**

**1 TBSP WATER**

---

1. Steam the peaches over a medium-high heat for 15 minutes.
2. Add to a food processor with the rest of the ingredients until puréed.
3. Serve right away or store in a sealable container in the fridge for 2-3 days.
4. Alternatively store in an ice cube tray and pop out to thaw before you need it.

Per serving: Calories: 6; Fat: 0g (Saturated Fat: 0g); Carbohydrates: 1g; Fiber: 0g; Sugar: 1g; Sodium: 31mg; Protein: 0g

# APRICOT CHUTNEY

**SERVES 10  /  PREP TIME: 5 MINUTES  /  COOK TIME: 15 MINUTES**

Great with crackers and low fat cheese.

---

**5 RIPE APRICOTS, PEELED**

**1/2 TSP CUMIN, GRATED**

**1/2 TSP HONEY**

**1 TBSP WATER**

---

1. Steam the apricots over a medium-high heat for 15 minutes.
2. Add to a food processor with the rest of the ingredients until puréed.
3. Serve right away or store in a sealable container in the fridge for 2-3 days.
4. Alternatively store in an ice cube tray and pop out to thaw before you need it.

Per serving: Calories: 17; Fat: 0g (Saturated Fat: 0g); Carbohydrates: 4g; Fiber: 1g; Sugar: 3g; Sodium: 56mg; Protein: 0g

# PUMPKIN PURÉE

SERVES 10 / PREP TIME: 10 MINUTES / COOK TIME: 30 MINUTES

Add to your favorite meal or eat as a snack.

---

4 CUPS PUMPKIN, PEELED AND CUBED

1 TSP NUTMEG

1 TSP STEVIA

4 CUPS VEGETABLE STOCK

---

1. Add the pumpkin to a large pot with the other ingredients over a medium-high heat for 30 minutes or until very soft.
2. Add to a food processor until puréed.
3. Serve right away or store in a sealable container in the fridge for 2-3 days.
4. Alternatively store in an ice cube tray and pop out to thaw before you need it.

Per serving: Calories: 23; Fat: 0g (Saturated Fat: 0g); Carbohydrates: 3g; Fiber: 0g; Sugar: 2g; Sodium: 7mg; Protein: 0g

# APPLE SAUCE

**SERVES 12  /  PREP TIME: 5 MINUTES  /  COOK TIME: 10 MINUTES**

This apple sauce tastes delicious with pork, fish or dessert!

---

**3 APPLES, PEELED AND CHOPPED**

**1 TBSP SKIMMED MILK OR EQUIVALENT**

**1/2 TSP NUTMEG**

**1/2 TSP CINNAMON**

---

1. Steam the chopped apples over a steamer on a medium-high heat for 10 minutes.
2. Combine apples with the rest of the ingredients and blend in a food processor until smooth.
3. If you don't have a processor, cook for an extra 5 minutes and mash with a fork before passing through a sieve and adding the rest of the ingredients.
4. Serve right away or store in a sealable container in the fridge for 2-3 days.
5. Alternatively store in an ice cube tray and pop out to thaw before you need it.

Per serving: Calories: 36; Fat: 0g (Saturated Fat: 0g); Carbohydrates: 6.5g; Fiber: 1.25g; Sugar: 1.5g; Sodium: 0mg; Protein: 0g

# SMOOTHIES AND DRINKS

# TROPICAL SMOOTHIE

**SERVES 2 / PREP TIME: 5 MINUTES / COOK TIME: N/A**

Sooth symptoms with this healthy juice.

---

**1/3 FROZEN SPINACH**

**1/3 CUP CANNED PINEAPPLE, DICED**

**1 CUP SKIM MILK OR DAIRY FREE EQUIVALENT**

---

1. Add all of the ingredients to a blender until smooth.
2. Serve cold over ice if desired!

Per serving: Calories: 76; Fat: 0g (Saturated Fat: 0g); Carbohydrates: 12g; Fiber: 1g; Sugar: 9.5g; Sodium: 117.5mg; Protein: 5g

# SUPER JUICE

**SERVES 2 / PREP TIME: 5 MINUTES / COOK TIME: N/A**

Sooth symptoms with this healthy juice.

---

**1/4 CUP FROZEN COOKED SPINACH**

**1/4 CUP FROZEN COOKED KALE**

**1/4 CUP MANGO, CHOPPED**

**1/2 CUP WATER**

---

1. Add all of the ingredients to a blender until smooth.
2. Serve cold over ice if desired!

Per serving: Calories: 20; Fat: 0g (Saturated Fat: 0g); Carbohydrates: 4g; Fiber: 1g; Sugar: 3g; Sodium: 14mg; Protein: 1g

# ALMOND MILKSHAKE

**SERVES 2 / PREP TIME: 5 MINUTES / COOK TIME: NA**

Nutty milkshake!

---

**2 CUPS SKIMMED MILK OR EQUIVALENT**

**1 TBSP ALMOND BUTTER**

**1 FROZEN BANANA**

---

1. Add all ingredients to a blender.
2. Blend until smooth.

Per serving: Calories: 190; Fat: 5g (Saturated Fat: 0g); Carbohydrates: 15g; Fiber: 0g; Sugar: 14g; Sodium: 130mg; Protein: 10g

# HOMEMADE RICE MILK

**SERVES 4 / PREP TIME: 5 MINUTES / COOK TIME: N/A**

Use as a replacement for cow's milk.

---

**3 CUPS COOKED WHITE RICE**

**12 CUPS WATER**

**1 TSP STEVIA**

**1 TSP VANILLA EXTRACT**

---

1. Add the ingredients to a blender or food processor and blend for 5 minutes until smooth.
2. Use right away or store in the fridge for 2-3 days.

Per serving: Calories: 150; Fat: 0g (Saturated Fat: 0g); Carbohydrates: 40g; Fiber: 0g; Sugar: 0g; Sodium: 0mg; Protein: 3g

# HOMEMADE ALMOND MILK

**SERVES 6  /  PREP TIME: 15 MINUTES / COOK TIME: N/A**

Another substitute for cow's milk.

---

**1/2 CUPS RAW ALMONDS**

**9 CUPS WATER**

**1 TSP STEVIA**

**1 TSP VANILLA EXTRACT**

---

1. Place almonds in a bowl with 3 cups water and allow to soak for 10-12 hours (overnight works well).
2. Drain and add the almonds to a food processor or blender.
3. Now add the 6 cups water to the blender and the stevia and vanilla extract for 5 minutes.
4. Use muslin over a fine sieve to strain the almond milk.
5. Squeeze out the muslin to get as much milk as possible.
6. Use right away or store in the fridge for 2-3 days.

Per serving: Calories: 69; Fat: 5g (Saturated Fat: 0g); Carbohydrates: 2g; Fiber: 1g; Sugar: 0g; Sodium: 0mg; Protein: 2g

# STRAWBERRY MILKSHAKE

**SERVES 4 / PREP TIME: 5 MINUTES / COOK TIME: N/A**

Delicious fruit drink!

---

**1 CUP CANNED STRAWBERRIES**

**1/4 CUP COOKED AND FROZEN SPINACH**

**2 CUPS ALMOND/SKIM MILK**

**1 TSP RAW HONEY**

---

1. Blend all ingredients in a food processor until smooth and then strain through a sieve to remove seeds and pips.
2. Serve over ice.

Per serving: Calories: 43; Fat: 5g (Saturated Fat: 0g); Carbohydrates: 7g; Fiber: 2g; Sugar: 3g; Sodium: 7mg; Protein: 2g

# PINEAPPLE & COCONUT SHAKE

**SERVES 4 / PREP TIME: 5 MINUTES / COOK TIME: NA**

Tropical and creamy.

---

**1/4 CUP FROZEN PINEAPPLE**

**1/4 CUP LIGHT COCONUT MILK**

**1 FROZEN BANANA**

---

1. Blend all ingredients in a food processor until smooth and then strain through a sieve to remove seeds and pips.
2. Serve over ice.

Per serving: Calories: 65; Fat: 1g (Saturated Fat: 1g); Carbohydrates: 13g; Fiber: 1g; Sugar: 8g; Sodium: 15mg; Protein: 1g

# GINGERBREAD LATTE

**SERVES 4 / PREP TIME: 5 MINUTES / COOK TIME: 5 MINUTES**

Warming and soothing for the stomach.

---

**2 CUPS ALMOND MILK**

**1 TSP GINGER, GRATED**

**1/2 TSP CINNAMON**

**1 TSP STEVIA**

---

1. Heat the milk in a small pot over a medium-high heat until it bubbles.
2. Add the ginger and cinnamon and allow to simmer on low for a further 5 minutes.
3. Remove from the heat and pour into your favorite mugs.
4. Stir in stevia if desired.

Per serving: Calories: 24; Fat: 2.5g (Saturated Fat: 2.5g); Carbohydrates: 0g; Fiber:1g; Sugar: 0g; Sodium: 2.5mg; Protein: 2g

# MOROCCAN MINT TEA

**SERVES 2 / PREP TIME: 5-10 MINUTES / COOK TIME: N/A**

Great for gastroparesis.

---

**2 CUPS BOILING WATER**

**1/4 CUP FRESH MINT/PEPPERMINT**

---

1. Pour the boiling water over the mint and allow to steep for 5-10 minutes.
2. Strain through a tea-strainer or sieve to serve.
3. If you have a tea pot, simply add mint and water to the tea pot and pour!
4. Add a little stevia if you like it sweet.

Per serving: Calories: 5; Fat: 0g (Saturated Fat: 0g); Carbohydrates: 1g; Fiber: 1g; Sugar: 0g; Sodium: 3mg; Protein: 0g

# BERRY DELIGHT

**SERVES 3 / PREP TIME: 5 MINUTES / COOK TIME: N/A**

Full of antioxidants!

---

**1/4 CUP FROZEN COOKED SPINACH**

**1/4 CUP FROZEN RASPBERRIES/ BLUEBERRIES**

**2 CUPS WATER**

**1/2 FROZEN BANANA**

---

1. Blend all ingredients in a food processor until smooth and then strain through a sieve to remove seeds and pips.
2. Serve over ice.

Per serving: Calories: 52; Fat: 3g (Saturated Fat: 2g); Carbohydrates: 6g; Fiber: 1g; Sugar: 3g; Sodium: 12mg; Protein: 1g

# VIRGIN BLOODY MARY

**SERVES 4 / PREP TIME: 10 MINUTES / COOK TIME: N/A**

A quick pick-me-up

---

**1 CUP HOMEMADE TOMATO SAUCE**

**3 CUPS WATER**

**1/4 CUP COOKED FROZEN SPINACH**

---

1. Blend all ingredients in a food processor until smooth and then strain through a sieve to remove seeds and pips.
2. Serve over ice.

Per serving: Calories: 42.5; Fat: 0.5g (Saturated Fat: 0g); Carbohydrates: 2.5g; Fiber: 1g; Sugar: 0g; Sodium: 80mg; Protein: 0g

# DESSERTS

# GRANDMA'S POACHED APPLES

**SERVES 2 / PREP TIME: 5 MINUTES / COOK TIME: 25 MINUTES**

Delicious!

---

**2 SMALL APPLES, PEELED, CORED AND HALVED**

**2 CLOVES**

**1 TSP CINNAMON**

**1 TBSP FAT FREE GREEK YOGURT**

---

1. Add the apples, cloves and cinnamon to a pot of water over a medium heat and simmer for 20-25 minutes or until apples are soft.
2. Serve hot with a helping of yogurt.

Per serving: Calories:35; Fat: 0g (Saturated Fat: 0g); Carbohydrates: 9g; Fiber: 2g; Sugar: 6g; Sodium: 4mg; Protein: 1g

# MANGO & PINEAPPLE SORBET

**SERVES 4  /  PREP TIME: Overnight  /  COOK TIME: NA**

Cold, sweet and refreshing.

---

**1 CAN MANGO PIECES IN SYRUP**

**1 CAN PINEAPPLE PIECES IN SYRUP**

---

1. Add the fruit pieces and syrup to a sealable container or plastic sandwich bag.
2. Freeze overnight and then remove and place in hot water to allow fruit to start thawing.
3. Add to a food processor until smooth.
4. Add to a sealable container and place in the freezer for at least 1 hour.
5. Remove from the freezer 5 minutes before serving.

Per serving: Calories: 40; Fat: 0g (Saturated Fat: 0g); Carbohydrates: 10g; Fiber: 1g; Sugar: 8g; Sodium: 0mg; Protein: 5g

# FROZEN YOGURT & BERRIES

**SERVES 4 / PREP TIME: 2-3 HOURS / COOK TIME: 10 MINUTES**

Frozen yogurt is simply delicious.

---

**2 CUPS NON-FAT GREEK YOGURT**

**1 CUP FROZEN BLACKBERRIES/
RASPBERRIES/BLUEBERRIES**

**1 TBSP RAW HONEY**

---

1. Add the berries to a small pot with 1/4 cup water over a low to medium heat.
2. Allow to simmer for 10 minutes or until fruit is very soft.
3. Strain through a sieve and allow to cool.
4. Stir through your yogurt and mix in the honey.
5. Add to a sealable container and place in the freezer for 2-3 hours. Stir every hour.
6. Remove and serve.

Per serving: Calories: 213; Fat: 5g (Saturated Fat: 3g); Carbohydrates: 20g; Fiber: 1g; Sugar: 13g; Sodium: 140mg; Protein: 23g

# CINNAMON & HONEY DOUGH BALLS

**SERVES 12 / PREP TIME: 15 MINUTES / COOK TIME: 15 MINUTES**

Enjoy!

---

- 1 TBSP STEVIA
- 1/2 TSP CINNAMON
- 1 TBSP RAW HONEY
- 1 SMALL EGG
- 2 TBSP SKIM MILK OR EQUIVALENT
- 3/4 CUP WHITE FLOUR (GF IF NEEDED)

- 1 TSP BAKING POWDER
- 1 TSP SUGAR
- 1 TBSP UNSALTED BUTTER
- 1 TSP WATER

---

1. Preheat the oven to 375°f/190°c/Gas Mark 5.
2. Spray a baking sheet with cooking spray or lightly grease with butter.
3. Mix together stevia and cinnamon.
4. In a separate bowl mix together the egg and milk.
5. In another bowl, mix the flour, baking powder, sugar, and butter. Rub together with your fingers until a breadcrumb consistency is reached.
6. Add the milk mixture to the breadcrumb mixture and mix well.
7. Onto a lightly floured surface, roll out your dough with a rolling pin until roughly 5cm thick.
8. Brush with a little extra milk and dust with the cinnamon mixture from earlier. Add a little water if necessary.
9. Divide dough into 12 and roll into balls.
10. Add to the baking sheet, leaving at least 1inch gap between each dough ball.
11. Bake for 12-15 minutes or until your knife pulls out clean from the centre.

Per serving: Calories: 26; Fat: 2g (Saturated Fat: 1g); Carbohydrates: 3g; Fiber: 0g; Sugar: 3g; Sodium: 157mg; Protein: 0g

# APPLE CINNAMON & HONEY CHIPS

**SERVES 8 / PREP TIME: 5 MINUTES / COOK TIME: 40 MINUTES**

Healthy apple chips.

---

**1 TSP UNSALTED BUTTER**

**2 APPLES, PEELED AND SLICED**

**1 TBSP HONEY**

**1 TSP NUTMEG**

---

1. Preheat the oven to 350°f/170°c/Gas Mark 4.
2. Lightly grease a baking tray with the butter.
3. Layer the apple slices and pour over the honey - toss to coat.
4. Sprinkle over the nutmeg and place in the oven for 30-40 minutes or until nice and crispy.

Per serving: Calories: 32; Fat: 0.5g (Saturated Fat: 0.5g); Carbohydrates: 7g; Fiber: 1g; Sugar: 6g; Sodium: 2.5mg; Protein: 2.5g

# POACHED PEARS

**SERVES 4 / PREP TIME: 5 MINUTES / COOK TIME: 25 MINUTES**

Delicious!

---

**2 WHOLE PEARS, PEELED**

**2 CLOVES**

**1 TSP NUTMEG**

**1 TBSP LOW-FAT GREEK YOGURT**

---

1. Add the pears, cloves and nutmeg to a pot of water over a medium heat and simmer for 20-25 minutes or until pears are soft.
2. Serve hot with a helping of yogurt.

Per serving: Calories: 39; Fat: 0g (Saturated Fat: 0g); Carbohydrates: 9g; Fiber: 1g; Sugar: 8g; Sodium: 4mg; Protein: 1g

# ALMOND CREAM

**SERVES 16 / PREP TIME: 5 MINUTES / COOK TIME: 10 MINUTES**

A tasty cream.

---

**1 CUP ALMOND MEAL**

**2 TBSP STEVIA**

**2 TBSP FLOUR**

**1/4 CUP ALMOND MILK**

**2 TBSP UNSALTED BUTTER**

**2 EGGS**

**1 TSP ALCOHOL FREE VANILLA EXTRACT**

---

1. Add the almond meal, stevia and flour to a food processor and blend until a paste is formed.
2. Add the almond milk and butter and blend for 2 minutes.
3. Now add the eggs one at a time and then the vanilla for 1 minute.
4. Heat in a pot over a medium heat for 5 minutes.
5. Serve as an addition to stewed fruits.

Per serving: Calories: 60; Fat: 5g (Saturated Fat: 1.5g); Carbohydrates: 2g; Fiber: 1g; Sugar: 2.5g; Sodium: 9mg; Protein: 2g

# PEACHES & CUSTARD

**SERVES 8 / PREP TIME: 5 MINUTES / COOK TIME: 50 MINUTES**

Yum!

---

| | |
|---|---|
| **8 EGGS** | **8 RAMEKINS** |
| **4 CUPS RICE MILK** | |
| **1/2 CUP HONEY** | |
| **1 CUP CANNED PEELED PEACHES** | |

---

1. Preheat the oven to 350°f/170°c/Gas Mark 4.
2. Beat the eggs in a mixing bowl.
3. Heat the rice milk and honey in a pot on a medium-high heat until bubbling (stir throughout).
4. Whilst stirring, gradually add 3 tablespoons of the hot milk into the beaten eggs.
5. Pour this mixture back into the pot with the rest of the milk (stir throughout).
6. Bring back to the boil whilst stirring for 5 minutes or until starting to thicken.
7. Add the peach slices to the base of each ramekin.
8. Pour mixture into 8 ramekins and add these to a baking dish.
9. Pour boiling water around the ramekins and place in the oven for 40 minutes.
10. Remove and allow to cool.
11. Serve!

Per serving: Calories: 256; Fat: 10g (Saturated Fat: 3g); Carbohydrates: 26g; Fiber: 1g; Sugar: 4g; Sodium: 127mg; Protein: 13g

# PUMPKIN PIE

**SERVES 8 / PREP TIME: 10 MINUTES / COOK TIME: 55 MINUTES**

Autumnal treat.

---

3/4 CUP SUGAR

1 TSP CINNAMON

1/4 TSP GROUND CLOVES

2 EGGS

2 TSP ALCOHOL FREE VANILLA EXTRACT

1/2 CUP PUMPKIN PURÉE

2 CUPS SKIM MILK OR EQUIVALENT

---

1. Preheat the oven to 425°f.
2. Mix the sugar and spices.
3. In a separate bowl, beat the eggs.
4. Mix the vanilla and pumpkin purée into the eggs.
5. Add the milk to the egg mixture before mixing in the spices.
6. Pour into a pie dish and bake in the oven for 15 minutes.
7. Reduce the temperature to 350°f/170°c/Gas Mark 4 and continue to bake for 40 minutes or until your knife comes out clean from the centre.
8. Remove and allow to cool slightly before serving.

Per serving: Calories: 122; Fat: 1g (Saturated Fat: 0.5g); Carbohydrates: 24g; Fiber: 1g; Sugar: 22.5g; Sodium: 119mg; Protein: 4g

# CONVERSION TABLES

Volume

| Imperial | Metric |
|---|---|
| 1 tbsp | 15ml |
| 2 fl oz | 55 ml |
| 3 fl oz | 75 ml |
| 5 fl oz (¼ pint) | 150 ml |
| 10 fl oz (½ pint) | 275 ml |
| 1 pint | 570 ml |
| 1 ¼ pints | 725 ml |
| 1 ¾ pints | 1 litre |
| 2 pints | 1.2 litres |
| 2½ pints | 1.5 litres |
| 4 pints | 2.25 litres |

Oven temperatures

| Gas Mark | Fahrenheit | Celsius |
|---|---|---|
| 1/4 | 225 | 110 |
| 1/2 | 250 | 130 |
| 1 | 275 | 140 |
| 2 | 300 | 150 |
| 3 | 325 | 170 |
| 4 | 350 | 180 |
| 5 | 375 | 190 |
| 6 | 400 | 200 |
| 7 | 425 | 220 |
| 8 | 450 | 230 |
| 9 | 475 | 240 |

Weight

| Imperial | Metric |
|---|---|
| ½ oz | 10 g |
| ¾ oz | 20 g |
| 1 oz | 25 g |
| 1½ oz | 40 g |
| 2 oz | 50 g |
| 2½ oz | 60 g |
| 3 oz | 75 g |
| 4 oz | 110 g |
| 4½ oz | 125 g |
| 5 oz | 150 g |
| 6 oz | 175 g |
| 7 oz | 200 g |
| 8 oz | 225 g |
| 9 oz | 250 g |
| 10 oz | 275 g |
| 12 oz | 350 g |

# BIBLIOGRAPHY

Olausson, E.A., Störsrud, S., Grundin, H., Isaksson, M., Attvall, S. and Simrén, M. (2014) 'A small particle size diet reduces upper gastrointestinal symptoms in patients with diabetic Gastroparesis: A Randomized controlled trial', The American Journal of Gastroenterology, 109(3), pp. 375–385. doi: 10.1038/ajg.2013.453. Garrick, R. (2008) 'Prevalence of chronic kidney disease in the United States', Yearbook of Medicine, 2008, pp. 215–217.

EMRAL, R. (2002) 'DIABETIC GASTROPARESIS (GASTROPARESIS DIABETICORUM)', Journal of Ankara Medical School, , pp. 001–008

PATRICK, A. and EPSTEIN, O. (2008) 'Review article: Gastroparesis', Alimentary Pharmacology & Therapeutics, 27(9), pp. 724–740.

Homko, C.J., Duffy, F., Friedenberg, F.K., Boden, G. and Parkman, H.P. (2015) 'Effect of dietary fat and food consistency on gastroparesis symptoms in patients with gastroparesis', Neurogastroenterology & Motility, 27(4), pp. 501–508

Nusrat, S. and Bielefeldt, K. (2012) 'Gastroparesis on the rise: Incidence vs awareness?', Neurogastroenterology & Motility, 25(1), pp. 16–22

Gastroparesis (2016) Available at: https://www.niddk.nih.gov/health-information/health-topics/digestive-diseases/gastroparesis/Pages/facts.aspx (Accessed: 6 September 2016).

American (2016) Gastroparesis. Available at: http://patients.gi.org/topics/gastroparesis/ (Accessed: 6 September 2016).

Staff, M.C. (2014) 'Gastroparesis definition', Mayoclinic, .

# INDEX

Made in the USA
San Bernardino, CA
08 April 2018